Medifocus Guidebook on:

Reflex Sympathetic Dystrophy

Last Update: 18 March 2014

Medifocus.com, Inc.

11529 Daffodil Lane
Suite 200
Silver Spring, MD 20902

www.medifocus.com

(800) 965-3002

MediFocus Guide #NR015

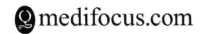

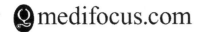

How To Use This Medifocus Guidebook

Before you start to review your *Guidebook*, it would be helpful to familiarize yourself with the organization and content of the information that is included in the Guidebook. Your *MediFocus Guidebook* is organized into the following five major sections.

- **Section 1: Background Information** - This section provides detailed information about the organization and content of the *Guidebook* including tips and suggestions for conducting additional research about the condition.

- **Section 2: The Intelligent Patient Overview** - This section is a comprehensive overview of the condition and includes important information about the cause of the disease, signs and symptoms, how the condition is diagnosed, the treatment options, quality of life issues, and questions to ask your doctor.

- **Section 3: Guide to the Medical Literature** - This section opens the door to the latest cutting-edge research and clinical advances recently published in leading medical journals. It consists of an extensive, focused selection of journal article references with links to the PubMed abstracts (summaries) of the articles. PubMed is the U.S. National Library of Medicine's database of references and abstracts from more than 4,500 medical and scientific articles published worldwide.

- **Section 4: Centers of Research** - This section is a unique directory of doctors, researchers, hospitals, medical centers, and research institutions with specialized interest and, in many cases, clinical expertise in the management of patients with the condition. You can use the "Centers of Research" directory to contact, consults, or network with leading experts in the field and to locate a hospital or medical center that can help you.

- **Section 5: Tips for Finding and Choosing a Doctor** - This section of your *Guidebook* offers important tips for how to find physicians as well as suggestions for how to make informed choices about choosing a doctor who is right for you.

- **Section 6: Directory of Organizations** - This section of your *Guidebook* is a directory of select disease organizations and support groups that are in the business of helping patients and their families by providing access to information, resources, and services. Many of these organizations can answer your questions, enable you to network with other patients, and help you find a doctor in your geographical area who specializes in managing your condition.

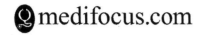

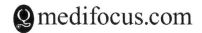 medifocus.com

Disclaimer

Medifocus.com, Inc. serves only as a clearinghouse for medical health information and does not directly or indirectly practice medicine. Any information provided by *Medifocus.com, Inc.* is intended solely for educating our clients and should not be construed as medical advice or guidance, which should always be obtained from a licensed physician or other health-care professional. As such, the client assumes full responsibility for the appropriate use of the medical and health information contained in the Guidebook and agrees to hold *Medifocus.com, Inc.* and any of its third-party providers harmless from any and all claims or actions arising from the clients' use or reliance on the information contained in this Guidebook. Although *Medifocus.com, Inc.* makes every reasonable attempt to conduct a thorough search of the published medical literature, the possibility always exists that some significant articles may be missed.

Copyright

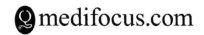

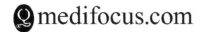
medifocus.com

Table of Contents

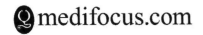

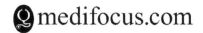

1 - Background Information

Introduction

Chronic or life-threatening illnesses can have a devastating impact on both the patient and the family. In today's new world of medicine, many consumers have come to realize that they are the ones who are primarily responsible for their own health care as well as for the health care of their loved ones.

When facing a chronic or life-threatening illness, you need to become an educated consumer in order to make an informed health care decision. Essentially that means finding out everything about the illness - the treatment options, the doctors, and the hospitals - so that you can become an educated health care consumer and make the tough decisions. In the past, consumers would go to a library and read everything available about a particular illness or medical condition. In today's world, many turn to the Internet for their medical information needs.

The first sites visited are usually the well known health "portals" or disease organizations and support groups which contain a general overview of the condition for the layperson. That's a good start but soon all of the basic information is exhausted and the need for more advanced information still exists. What are the latest "cutting-edge" treatment options? What are the results of the most up-to-date clinical trials? Who are the most notable experts? Where are the top-ranked medical institutions and hospitals?

The best source for authoritative medical information in the United States is the National Library of Medicine's medical database called PubMed, that indexes citations and abstracts (brief summaries) of over 7 million articles from more than 3,800 medical journals published worldwide. PubMed was developed for medical professionals and is the primary source utilized by health care providers for keeping up with the latest advances in clinical medicine.

A typical PubMed search for a specific disease or condition, however, usually retrieves hundreds or even thousands of "hits" of journal article citations. That's an avalanche of information that needs to be evaluated and transformed into truly useful knowledge. What are the most relevant journal articles? Which ones apply to your specific situation? Which articles are considered to be the most authoritative - the ones your physician would rely on in making clinical decisions? This is where *Medifocus.com* provides an effective solution.

Medifocus.com has developed an extensive library of *MediFocus Guidebooks* covering a wide spectrum of chronic and life threatening diseases. Each *MediFocus Guidebook* is a high quality, up- to-date digest of "professional-level" medical information consisting of the most relevant citations and abstracts of journal articles published in authoritative, trustworthy medical journals. This information represents the latest advances known to modern medicine for the treatment and management of the condition, including published results from clinical trials. Each *Guidebook* also includes a valuable index of leading authors and medical institutions as well as a directory of disease organizations and support groups. *MediFocus Guidebooks* are reviewed, revised and updated every 4-months to ensure that you receive the latest and most up-to-date information about the specific condition.

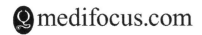medifocus.com

About Your MediFocus Guidebook

Introduction

Your *MediFocus Guidebook* is a valuable resource that represents a comprehensive synthesis of the most up-to-date, advanced medical information published about the condition in well-respected, trustworthy medical journals. It is the same type of professional-level information used by physicians and other health-care professionals to keep abreast of the latest developments in biomedical research and clinical medicine. The *Guidebook* is intended for patients who have a need for more advanced, in-depth medical information than is generally available to consumers from a variety of other resources. The primary goal of a *MediFocus Guidebook* is to educate patients and their families about their treatment options so that they can make informed health-care decisions and become active participants in the medical decision making process.

The *Guidebook* production process involves a team of experienced medical research professionals with vast experience in researching the published medical literature. This team approach to the development and production of the *MediFocus Guidebooks* is designed to ensure the accuracy, completeness, and clinical relevance of the information. The *Guidebook* is intended to serve as a basis for a more meaningful discussion between patients and their health-care providers in a joint effort to seek the most appropriate course of treatment for the disease.

Guidebook Organization and Content

Section 1 - Background Information
This section provides detailed information about the organization and content of the *Guidebook* including tips and suggestions for conducting additional research about the condition.

Section 2 - The Intelligent Patient Overview
This section of your *MediFocus Guidebook* represents a detailed overview of the disease or condition specifically written from the patient's perspective. It is designed to satisfy the basic informational needs of consumers and their families who are confronted with the illness and are facing difficult choices. Important aspects which are addressed in "The Intelligent Patient" section include:

- The etiology or cause of the disease
- Signs and symptoms
- How the condition is diagnosed

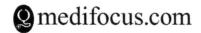

- The current standard of care for the disease
- Treatment options
- New developments
- Important questions to ask your health care provider

Section 3 - Guide to the Medical Literature

This is a roadmap to important and up-to-date medical literature published about the condition from authoritative, trustworthy medical journals. This is the same information that is used by physicians and researchers to keep up with the latest developments and breakthroughs in clinical medicine and biomedical research. A broad spectrum of articles is included in each *MediFocus Guidebook* to provide information about standard treatments, treatment options, new clinical developments, and advances in research. To facilitate your review and analysis of this information, the articles are grouped by specific categories. A typical *MediFocus Guidebook* usually contains one or more of the following article groupings:

- *Review Articles:* Articles included in this category are broad in scope and are intended to provide the reader with a detailed overview of the condition including such important aspects as its cause, diagnosis, treatment, and new advances.

- *General Interest Articles:* These articles are broad in scope and contain supplementary information about the condition that may be of interest to select groups of patients.

- *Drug Therapy:* Articles that provide information about the effectiveness of specific drugs or other biological agents for the treatment of the condition.

- *Surgical Therapy:* Articles that provide information about specific surgical treatments for the condition.

- *Clinical Trials:* Articles in this category summarize studies which compare the safety and efficacy of a new, experimental treatment modality to currently available standard treatments for the condition. In many cases, clinical trials represent the latest advances in the field and may be considered as being on the "cutting edge" of medicine. Some of these experimental treatments may have already been incorporated into clinical practice.

The following information is provided for each of the articles referenced in this section of your *MediFocus Guidebook:*

- Article title

medifocus.com

- Author Name(s)
- Institution where the study was done
- Journal reference (Volume, page numbers, year of publication)
- Link to Abstract (brief summary of the actual article)

Linking to Abstracts: Most of the medical journal articles referenced in this section of your *MediFocus Guidebook* include an abstract (brief summary of the actual article) that can be accessed online via the National Library of Medicine's PubMed® database. You can easily access the individual article abstracts online by entering the individual URL address for a particular article into your web browser, or by going to the URL listed on the bottom of each page of this section.

Section 4 - Centers of Research

We've compiled a unique directory of doctors, researchers, medical centers, and research institutions with specialized research interest, and in many cases, clinical expertise in the management of the specific medical condition. The "Centers of Research" directory is a valuable resource for quickly identifying and locating leading medical authorities and medical institutions within the United States and other countries that are considered to be at the forefront in clinical research and treatment of the condition.

Inclusion of the names of specific doctors, researchers, hospitals, medical centers, or research institutions in this *Guidebook* does not imply endorsement by Medifocus.com, Inc. or any of its affiliates. Consumers are encouraged to conduct additional research to identify health-care professionals, hospitals, and medical institutions with expertise in providing specific medical advice, guidance, and treatment for this condition.

Section 5 - Tips on Finding and Choosing a Doctor

One of the most important decisions confronting patients who have been diagnosed with a serious medical condition is finding and choosing a qualified physician who will deliver high-level, quality medical care in accordance with curently accepted guidelines and standards of care. Finding the "best" doctor to manage your condition, however, can be a frustrating and time-consuming experience unless you know what you are looking for and how to go about finding it. This section of your Guidebook offers important tips for how to find physicians as well as suggestions for how to make informed choices about choosing a doctor who is right for you.

Section 6 - Directory of Organizations

This section of your *Guidebook* is a directory of select disease organizations and support groups that are in the business of helping patients and their families by providing access to information, resources, and services. Many of these organizations can answer your questions, enable you to network with other patients, and help you find a doctor in your

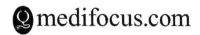

geographical area who specializes in managing your condition.

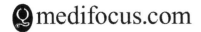 medifocus.com

Ordering Full-Text Articles

After reviewing your *MediFocus Guidebook*, you may wish to order the full-text copy of some of the journal article citations that are referenced in the *Guidebook*. There are several options available for obtaining full-text copies of journal articles, however, with the exception of obtaining the article yourself by visiting a nearby medical library, most involve a fee to cover the costs of photocopying, delivering, and paying the copyright royalty fees set by the individual publishers of medical journals.

This section of your *MediFocus Guidebook* provides some basic information about how you can go about obtaining full-text copies of journal articles from various fee-based document delivery resources.

Commercial Document Delivery Services

There are numerous commercial document delivery companies that provide full-text photocopying and delivery services to the general public. The costs may vary from company to company so it is worth your while to carefully shop-around and compare prices. Some of these commercial document delivery services enable you to order articles directly online from the company's web site. You can locate companies that provide document delivery services by typing the key words "document delivery" into any major Internet search engine.

National Library of Medicine's "Loansome Doc" Document Retrieval Services

The National Library of Medicine (NLM), located in Bethesda, Maryland, offers full-text photocopying and delivery of journal articles through its on-line service known as "Loansome Doc". To learn more about how you can order articles using "Loansome Doc", please visit the NLM web site at:
http://www.nlm.nih.gov/pubs/factsheets/loansome_doc.html

Participating "Loansome Doc" Libraries: United States

In the United States there are approximately 250 medical libraries that participate in the National Library of Medicine's "Loansome Doc" document retrieval and delivery services for the general public. Please note that each participating library sets its own policies and

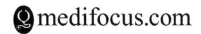
charges for providing document retrieval services. To order full-text copies of articles, simply contact a participating "Loansome Doc" medical library in your geographical area and ask to speak with one of the reference librarians. They can answer all of your questions including fees, delivery options, and turn-around time.

Here is how to find a participating "Loansome Doc" library in the U.S. that provides article retrieval services for the general public:

- **United States** - Contact a Regional Medical Library at 1-800-338-7657 (Monday - Friday; 8:30 AM - 5:30 PM). They will provide information about libraries in your area with which you may establish an account for the "Loansome Doc" service.

- **Canada** - Contact the Canada Institute for Scientific and Technical Information (CISTI) at 1-800-668-1222 for information about libraries in your area.

International MEDLARS Centers

If you reside outside the United States, you can obtain copies of medical journal articles through one of several participating International Medical Literature Analysis and Retrieval Systems (MEDLARS) Centers that provide "Loansome Doc" services in over 20 major countries. International MEDLARS Centers can be found in some of these countries: Australia, Canada, China, Egypt, France, Germany, Hong Kong, India, Israel, Italy, Japan, Korea, Kuwait, Mexico, Norway, Russia, South Africa, Sweden, and the United Kingdom. A complete listing of International MEDLARS Centers, including locations and telephone contact information can be viewed at:
http://www.nlm.nih.gov/pubs/factsheets/intlmedlars.html

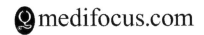
NOTES

Use this page for taking notes as you review your Guidebook

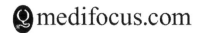
2 - The Intelligent Patient Overview

REFLEX SYMPATHETIC DYSTROPHY

Introduction to Reflex Sympathetic Dystrophy

What is Reflex Sympathetic Dystrophy?

Reflex sympathetic dystrophy (RSD), also known as *complex regional pain syndrome* (CRPS) *Type I*, is a chronic pain syndrome that can affect any part of the body; however, it occurs most frequently in the extremities - hands, feet, arms, legs, shoulders or knees. It has been recognized by many clinicians as a distinct clinical condition for over 100 years and has been known by various names including *algodystrophy*, *Sudeck's atrophy*, *causalgia* (now known as CRPS II), and *sympathetically-maintained pain*.

Reflex sympathetic dystrophy is characterized by:

- Severe, chronic pain often described as stinging or burning
- Sensory abnormalities such as *allodynia* (pain due to a stimulus which does not normally provoke pain) or *hyperesthesia* (increased sensitivity to stimuli)
- Motor impairment such as weakness, tremor, stiffness, or decreased range of motion
- *Edema* (tissue swelling) and *hyperhydrosis* (excessive sweating)
- Progressive *trophic* changes to skin, hair, nails, muscle, and bone (such as thinning of bones or changes in how hair and nails grow)
- Increasing dysfunction of the affected limb

Reflex sympathetic dystrophy causes great suffering and distress in most patients. In addition to severe pain, which in some people remains chronic and unremitting, patients may also experience serious physical disabilities and reduction in their quality of life leading to:

- Depression
- Fear
- Anxiety
- Anger

The syndrome of RSD is not well understood but it occurs most often after trauma such as

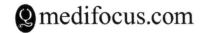
a bone fracture or surgery to an extremity. The trauma can also be very minor such as a splinter, sprained ankle, or following intravenous needle insertion. RSD can also occur following a serious medical condition such as a heart attack or stroke. In up to 25% of RSD patients, however, no apparent cause can be established with certainty. Although the symptoms and clinical features of RSD can vary from patient to patient, the one common cardinal feature that is shared by all patients is severe pain that is disproportionate to the original injury. Reflex sympathetic dystrophy does not exist in the absence of pain.

The perception of pain is a complex event and relates to physiological as well as psychological components. Usually pain is perceived immediately following a precipitating event such as trauma and, after the pain stimulus has been eliminated, the body returns to the previous state of being pain-free. When pain continues beyond an acceptable time period and/or appears to intensify, the pain is said to become *pathologic*. This is the essence of RSD. As the body responds for a prolonged time period to pathologic pain, it can cause permanent structural or functional changes within the affected extremity and, ultimately, in the central nervous system. Even within the variability of individual perception, tolerance, and response to pain, the pain of RSD is totally out of proportion to the precipitating event.

Although the term *reflex sympathetic dystrophy* has been used to describe the condition since the 1940s, it has recently come under scrutiny since it is misleading for several reasons, including:

- There is little evidence of involvement of a reflex mechanism
- Symptoms of RSD reflect a complicated interplay of several neurological systems, such as the peripheral and central nervous systems, not only the sympathetic nervous system
- Only a subset of patients respond to a treatment to reduce pain called a *sympathetic block* which interrupts the activity of the sympathetic nervous system, indicating that not all RSD pain is sympathetically mediated
- *Dystrophy* (degeneration of muscle or tissue) is present only in a subset of RSD patients (approximately 10%)

In response to these inconsistencies, the International Association for the Study of Pain (IASP) adopted the term *complex regional pain syndrome* (CRPS) in 1994 to describe a debilitating pain syndrome that develops after a relatively minor injury to an extremity (arm or leg) but lasts longer than the actual injury and is more severe than would otherwise be expected from such an injury. There are two types of CRPS:

- *CRPS Type I* - also known as *reflex sympathetic dystrophy* where the pain is not associated with any identifiable nerve injury
- *CRPS Type II* - also known as *causalgia* where the pain can be traced to a nerve

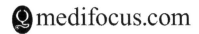

injury

Despite extensive research over the past several decades, researchers still do not understand clearly the underlying pathological mechanisms involved in the initiation and progression of RSD including:

- Why RSD develops in some people and not others
- Why RSD goes into remission for some people and not others
- Why some people experience recurrence of RSD
- What are the most effective treatments for RSD
- How to prevent RSD from occurring

What Causes Pain in Reflex Sympathetic Dystrophy?

The mechanism of action in reflex sympathetic dystrophy (RSD) is not well understood and is the subject of extensive debate. Much of the confusion is due to the fact that RSD is clearly not a condition caused exclusively by the sympathetic nervous system and many experts believe that there must be a more complex reaction occurring in response to precipitating events that cause RSD.

There are at least two possible origins of pain in RSD: *sympathetically-maintained pain* which is pain caused by some "malfunction" in the sympathetic nervous system, and *sympathetically-independent pain*.

Sympathetically-Maintained Pain

The sympathetic nervous system (SNS) regulates involuntary responses to stress such as increased heart rate and constriction of peripheral blood vessels as well as some of the body's initial response to any injury. Research indicates that the sympathetic nervous system also plays a role in neuropathic and inflammatory pain. In patients with RSD, there may be evidence of more widespread impairment of sympathetic nervous system function which is not necessarily limited to the affected extremity.

Until recently, it was thought that RSD was characterized by sympathetically-maintained pain where the SNS basically overreacted to an injury. Typically, after an injury occurs, the sympathetic nervous system is activated. It mobilizes the body's inflammatory response with the release of certain substances in order begin the process of healing the wound. The sympathetic response typically decreases within minutes or hours after the initial injury. When the inflammatory response continues unchecked, even when the stimulus is no longer present, the pain becomes sympathetically driven and the condition known as RSD develops. When treatment is directed towards interrupting the sympathetically-maintained

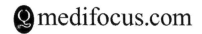

pain, the patient experiences relief from pain.

Sympathetically-Independent Pain

With *sympathetically-independent pain*, the pain is caused by a combination of factors that interact with the SNS, such as the peripheral and central nervous systems. Treatments directed towards the SNS do not bring relief to people experiencing this type of pain.

Reflex sympathetic dystrophy appears to be disorder involving a combination of the sympathetic nervous system in addition to peripheral, central, immune, or vascular systems. In effect, what may be happening with RSD is that a vicious cycle is created: the sympathetic response leads to chemical changes which then activate the response of other systems (e.g., central nervous system) which leads to more pain, which leads to more chemical changes, and so on.

Some evidence indicating the RSD is not exclusively related to the sympathetic nervous system includes:

- While some symptoms of RSD can be traced to the sympathetic nervous system, such as pain, or changes in sweating of the affected limb, other symptoms, such as warming of the limb, or swelling, are caused by substances released from other sources such as damaged blood vessels and not the sympathetic nervous system.

- Sympathectomy, a procedure which interrupts the flow of the sympathetic nervous system, is effective for individual patients; however larger clinical studies have shown the procedure to be no more effective than a placebo.

- The symptoms of RSD do not include those typically seen by an overactive sympathetic nervous system, such as an overactive thyroid and increased heart rate, or by an underactive sympathetic nervous system, such as decreased sweating, orthostatic hypertension (drop in blood pressure when changing positions), or ejaculation problems.

In short, it appears that the pain of RSD is not related to an overactive sympathetic nervous system, but rather, reflects a more global involvement including:

- Peripheral nervous system
- Sympathetic nervous system
- Central nervous system
- Vascular system
- Immune system
- Inflammatory responses

Risk Factors for Reflex Sympathetic Dystrophy

Several risk factors for the development of reflex sympathetic dystrophy (RSD) have been identified including:

- Trauma - Bone fracture, sprain, or other injury to the affected limb, often minor in nature, is considered the leading provocative event. Bone fractures account for up to 45-50% of cases of RSD.
- Surgery - RSD has been reported to occur following certain surgical procedures on the extremities such as carpal tunnel release surgery, knee arthroscopy, hip arthroplasty, amputation, or ankle arthrodesis (surgical fusion of the joint), and knee replacement surgery. It is estimated that up to 19% of patients with RSD have undergone knee replacement surgery.
- Cardiovascular events - Ischemic heart disease, heart attack, or stroke have been reported as risk factors for developing RSD. Estimates of RSD in stroke patients range from 12-60%.
- Neurological events - RSD may be seen as part of other neurological diseases such as carpal tunnel syndrome or pinched spinal nerves.
- Neoplasms - Certain types of cancers may produce a CRPS-like syndrome (e.g., lung cancer, breast cancer, and ovarian cancer).
- Age - Incidence of RSD is highest in people between the ages of 50-70 years old. The mean age of diagnosis reported in studies ranges between 46-52 years old.
- Gender - Adult females are affected at a rate three times higher than males.
- Genetic predisposition - It appears that people with RSD are more likely to have certain HLA tissue types than control groups, but the meaning of this finding is unclear. HLA stands for Human Leukocyte Antigens and they are proteins found on the surface of white blood cells.
- Incorrect immobilization of a limb - While immobilization may be necessary in certain situations, it could also become a precipitating factor in the development of RSD. Studies involving immobilization of limbs in healthy subjects resulted in symptoms identical with RSD, such as *trophic* changes, muscle stiffness or atrophy, changes in skin color and temperature, circulation problems to the affected limb, and pain when the casts were removed. Trophic changes are abnormalities of the skin, hair, nails, subcutaneous tissues and bone, caused by peripheral nerve injury.
- Poorly fitted casts or splints.

In approximately 10-25% of patients with reflex sympathetic dystrophy, no precipitating event can be identified. Sometimes because the trauma may have been so minor (e.g., a splinter), the patient does not recall the event or may not have been aware of it when it occurred.

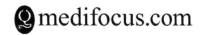

There is continuing discussion regarding the prevention of RSD following situations involving immobilization of a fracture or stroke. Some clinicians have suggested that certain precautions may offset or at least minimize the development of RSD if performed before or after surgery takes place. These include:

- Attention to pain prevention
- Early mobilization of the limb
- Prophylactic physical therapy
- Attention to properly fitted cast or splint

Recent research has shown an advantage to prescribing 500 mg. of vitamin C daily from the time of the fracture or precipitating event (such as surgery).

Incidence of Reflex Sympathetic Dystrophy

The incidence of reflex sympathetic dystrophy (RSD) in the general population is a subject of extensive debate since only two population-based studies have been published and their results varied widely. A study conducted in 2003 in the U.S. reported that the incidence of RSD was approximately five per 100,000 people annually, while a study completed in the Netherlands in 2006 reported a rate of approximately 26 people per 100,000 annually. If those standards were applied in the U.S. population, it would translate into approximately 50,000 new cases of RSD annually. Part of the reason for this wide discrepancy in the two studies is the lack of standardized criteria for the diagnosis of RSD.

Additional information about the incidence of RSD includes:

- Female-to-male ratio is approximately 4:1
- Median age of onset is approximately 46 - 52, but RSD can occur at any age
- Upper limbs are affected approximately twice as often as lower limbs
- Fracture is the most common trigger for RSD (46% of cases)
- There is a higher incidence of RSD around puberty
- In children, the ratio of *lower* limb involvement to *upper* limb is approximately 5:1 (opposite of adults)
- Recurrence of RSD may be higher for childhood-onset RSD than for adult-onset

Reflex Sympathetic Dystrophy in Children

Reflex sympathetic dystrophy (RSD) in children and adolescents is similar to that in adults except that in children there is a preponderance of the lower extremity over the upper extremity (especially the foot) and RSD most often occurs following minor trauma. RSD

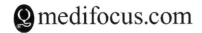
affects girls more than boys and the incidence is greatest at and just before puberty. It is more common among Caucasian children that among non-Caucasians.

For more information about RSD in children, please click on the following link: http://www.ncbi.nlm.nih.gov/pubmed/19143976

Reflex Sympathetic Dystrophy and Stroke

The incidence of reflex sympathetic dystrophy (RSD) in post-stroke patients is thought to be severely underdiagnosed. There are some reports that the incidence may be as high as 60% of patients. In this population, RSD is usually found in the upper extremity and is also known as *shoulder-hand syndrome*. It shares the same underlying problem encountered with most cases of RSD, namely immobilization of the limb.

In a study that appeared in the *International Journal of Rehabilitation and Research* in 2007, researchers reported that RSD developed in 48% of the 82 patients included in the study in the first 28 weeks following the stroke. They noted that the presence of RSD was significantly correlated with the presence of:

- Shoulder subluxation - a partial dislocation of the shoulder joint
- Spasticity of shoulder muscles
- Loss of range of motion in the shoulder joint
- Loss of muscle strength

To read more about the relationship between stroke and RSD, please click on the following link: http://www.ncbi.nlm.nih.gov/pubmed/17293718

Recurrence of Reflex Sympathetic Dystrophy

It has been estimated that the recurrence rate of reflex sympathetic dystrophy (RSD) in the same or another limb is 4-10% and that it recurs between three and twenty years after the initial event. Most cases of recurrence develop after a subsequent trauma or surgery. This has led some researchers to conclude that susceptibility to RSD recurrence may be increased after initial development of the condition. The recurrence rate of childhood-onset RSD is thought to be approximately 33%.

Does Reflex Sympathetic Dystrophy Spread?

Many patients report that RSD spreads from the location of the initial injury. Spreading may occur in three patterns:

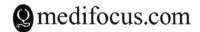

- *Contiguous spread* - This occurs in almost all patients and involves the gradual enlargement of the affected area.
- *Independent spread* - Signs and symptoms appear at distant sites not adjacent to the initial site of the injury. This pattern occurs in up to 70% of patients with RSD.
- *Mirror image spread* - Signs and symptoms appear in the same area on the opposite (contralateral) limb. This pattern occurs in up to 15% of patients.

The Reflex Sympathetic Dystrophy Syndrome Association (RSDSA) notes that spreading represents chronic changes that take place in the central nervous system or may represent overuse of the unaffected limb or may be related to some type of invasive procedure. The RSDSA notes that spreading of the pain in the same limb or region of the body is more likely to be related to a *myofascial pain syndrome*.

The *myofascia* is a layer of loose but strong connective tissue that covers all muscles. Myofascial pain is a soft tissue disorder that is typically localized to one area of the body. It is characterized by "trigger points" which are highly irritable spots in a particular area of muscle fiber that, when compressed, cause significant pain and tenderness in an area larger than the trigger point itself. When patients with RSD make adaptive adjustments to protect the painful limb, for example, by tightening or contracting the supporting muscles of the shoulder or neck to protect a painful hand, they cause changes at the myofascial level of the muscle as well. Or, when patients overuse the unaffected limb to compensate for the disability of the affected limb, the overworked or poorly conditioned muscles and myofascia are affected and can cause pain that affects not only that limb but can radiate to other parts of the body, such as the head, or chest. Thus, myofascial pain is complex in its pattern and not necessarily related to the original location. This may be interpreted by the patient as the sensation of "spreading".

The RSDSA estimates that between 60-80% of people suffering from RSD are affected by myofascial pain.

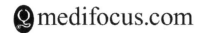
Diagnosis of Sympathetic Reflex Dystrophy

Significant controversy and confusion surrounds the diagnosis of reflex sympathetic dystrophy (RSD) due to several factors including:

- Lack of universal recognition of RSD as a medical diagnosis - Opinions among health care professionals range from dismissing or disregarding RSD as a legitimate diagnosis to considering it significantly underdiagnosed, especially in the early stage. A diagnosis is easier to reach in severe or advanced cases, by which time most patients are refractory (resistant) to therapy. Patients who reach a severe stage constitute a minority of those suffering from RSD.
- Lack of a "gold standard" regarding diagnostic criteria for RSD - Several different guidelines have been published and each differs in terms of the number of signs and symptoms which must be present in order to reach a diagnosis. To date, no diagnostic test has been validated for the diagnosis of RSD.
- Patients may be seen by different types of physicians for their symptoms (such as primary care physicians or orthopedists) who may not be familiar with RSD because they have not seen it often in their practice or they think RSD is a rare disease and so do not include it in the differential diagnosis.

Signs and Symptoms of Reflex Sympathetic Dystrophy

Reflex sympathetic dystrophy (RSD) is associated a wide range of symptoms, and except for pain, some but not all of the symptoms are required for establishing a diagnosis. Signs and symptoms include:

Sensory Involvement
- Pain - described as severe, deep, burning, and/or aching (up to 80% of patients)
- Allodynia - pain from innocuous, tactile stimulation of the skin, such as a light breeze or the touch of a feather (up to 65% of patients)
- *Tinel's sign* - severe pain following gentle tapping on the skin
- Sudden jolts of sharp pain - typically occur at *trigger points* on the involved limb (hyperirritable spots on the muscle)

Motor Involvement
- Decreased flexion of the affected limb that can lead to progressive loss of muscle mass or *wasting* (atrophy) and can result in contracture of the limb
- Reduced range of motion (up to 80% of patients)
- *Dystonia* which is slow movement or spasm in a group of muscles resulting in

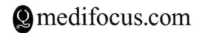

clenched fist, fingers that are flexed and fixed in position, contractures (severe muscles contractions), or clubfoot (up to 14% of patients)
- Weakness in the affected limb (up to 75% of patients)
- Tremor where the patient feels like the limb is jumping (up to 20% of patients)
- Neglect of the affected limb (ignoring the limb, disuse)
- Difficulty initiating movement
- Difficulty in maintaining movement (e.g., legs may buckle or an item may fall from the hand while holding it)

Trophic changes:
- Brittle nails which may grow faster or slower than the others (up to 20% of patients)
- Hair may grow in faster and/or curlier on the affected limb (up to 18% of patients)
- Smooth, glossy appearance to skin (up to 24% of patients)
- Patchy bone demineralization

Sudomotor (Sweat) Changes
- Increased sweating (hyperhydrosis)
- Asymmetry of sweating between the affected limb and the rest of the body (up to 53% of patients)

Vasomotor Changes
- Increase or decrease of skin temperature (up to 79% of patients)
- Changes in skin color of the affected limb, such as cyanosis (blue), red, or mottled color (up to 85% of patients)
- White patchy areas of skin
- Edema or swelling of the affected limb (up to 80% of patients)

Lower extremity RSD may initially be associated with inflammation and raised skin temperature of the affected area (indicating increased but nutrition-poor blood flow) and then progress to a cold stage which is associated with atrophy of the limb.

Psychological Changes
Psychological changes are common among people with RSD but they are not included in the diagnostic criteria. Psychological changes may include:

- Fear
- Anxiety
- Sense of suffering
- Anger
- Depression
- Failure to cope

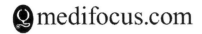

- Behavioral problems

Other Symptoms

Other symptoms which may be present in RSD include:

- Poor dentition - the increased sympathetic nervous system activity can cause poor nutritional blood flow to the jaw
- *Dissociation* - pain and swelling are present in one extremity but a movement disorder may be apparent on the contralateral (opposite) side.
- Visual blurring and difficulty focusing
- Rapid bone loss - the pathogenesis of this symptom is not clearly understood. It is thought that it may be due to either the immobilization of the affected limb or not being involved in weight-bearing activity while it is immobilized (such as lifting). However, the bone loss that occurs with RSD appears to be greater than would be expected if these two factors alone were the cause.
- Myofascial pain in the *proximal* joint of the area affected by RSD (for example with RSD of the hand, pain may be felt in the elbow). This symptom is commonly reported among patients with RSD.

Stages of Reflex Sympathetic Dystrophy

Some experts believe that there are three stages of reflex sympathetic dystrophy (RSD) that represent different clinical stages of the disease process. The progression of these stages has not, however, been validated by clinical studies and is the subject of ongoing debate. The three stages are as follows:

- Stage I usually lasts from one to three months after onset and is characterized by:

  - pain - the pain is severe, burning or throbbing and is localized to the limb
  - edema - swelling that is usually localized to the affected limb and may have a well demarcated edge
  - skin changes - skin in the area takes on a blue tinge in color and becomes cold and sweaty
  - skin begins to atrophy and becomes shiny
  - increased sweating (hyperhydrosis)
  - rapid hair growth
  - joint stiffness
  - muscle spasm
  - early evidence of osteoporosis (thin, weak bone more susceptible to fracture)

- Stage II lasts 3-6 months and is characterized by:

- intensifying pain
- swelling
- weak muscle tone
- hair may become coarse and may be followed by hair loss
- nails may grow faster or slower and may become brittle, spotty, or grooved
- joint stiffness worsens with further reduced range of motion
- bones begin to soften

- Stage III is characterized by:

  - unremitting pain that may involve the entire limb
  - sensory disturbance (e.g., allodynia)
  - marked muscle atrophy
  - severely limited mobility
  - significant increase of motor and trophic changes
  - irreversible changes of skin and bone
  - loss of function and stiffness of the limb
  - marked osteoporosis
  - involuntary contraction of muscles and tendons which may make limbs contorted. In the upper extremity, this may take the form of frozen shoulder or "claw hand"

Since there is considerable variability regarding the intensity and duration of symptoms, and the course of the disease seems to be so unpredictable among patients, the usefulness of classifying RSD by stages is under debate. In 2002, an article was published in *Pain* (vol. 95(1-2):119-24) in which the authors proposed an alternative means of identifying subgroups of RSD which would help to target treatment more effectively. These subgroups include:

- Relatively limited RSD where vasomotor symptoms predominate (skin color and temperature changes)
- Relatively limited RSD with predominance of neuropathic pain and sensory disturbances
- Florid RSD which is similar to "classic RSD" characterized by:

  - high levels of motor and trophic changes
  - changes related to disuse of the limb such as *osteopenia* (changes in calcium levels that is a precursor to osteoporosis and leads to increased risks such as fracture)
  - pain that is not necessarily a predominant symptom and may be of brief

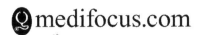

duration

Diagnostic Testing for Reflex Sympathetic Dystrophy

Currently, there is no single test for the diagnosis of reflex sympathetic dystrophy (RSD). Therefore, physicians use both subjective (patient history) and objective (physical examination) methods to establish a diagnosis. Imaging or other tests may be included to confirm the diagnosis or to rule out other conditions.

Patient History

In many cases, the patient's history reveals that a recent injury to the site (often minor in nature) or a surgical procedure preceded the onset of RSD symptoms. If a precipitating event can be identified after which the magnitude of pain and other symptoms significantly exceeds what would otherwise be expected from the initial event, RSD should be considered as part of the differential diagnosis. Often, the injury may be so slight (e.g., a splinter) that the patient does not recall ever having sustained it.

Physical Examination

The doctor conducts a physical examination to determine the presence and extent of symptoms reported by the patient which may include:

- Range of motion of the affected limb
- Allodynia (pain from a normally nonpainful stimulus) and hyperalgesia (increased sensitivity to pain) as a response to various stimuli
- Temperature or color changes
- Changes to hair, nails, or skin
- Evidence of edema
- Presence of the Tinel sign - To evoke the Tinel sign, the doctor holds up the limb above the horizontal plane and taps the area above the nerve suspected to be involved to see if the patient feels a tingling sensation or pain. If the test is positive, it may be an indication that the origin of the upper extremity RSD is a brachial plexus injury.

Some patients develop a tendency to "guard" the affected limb (also called "bracing") from painful situations such as being touched or bumped and they may not allow the physician to examine or manipulate the limb. As a result of this extreme disuse and neglect of the limb, the doctor may notice that the limb is no longer washed or cared for by the patient.

Imaging Studies

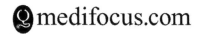

Imaging studies do not play a significant role in the diagnosis of RSD. They function more as a means of ruling out other medical conditions that may cause similar symptoms.

- X-ray - used often as a preliminary study that shows the mineralization status of the bone and also may be performed to track progression of RSD. Demineralization in RSD may increase over time due to disuse and ensuing loss of function of the affected limb. In general, the utility of X-rays in the diagnosis of RSD is limited.
- Bone Scintigraphy (bone scan) - Used since the 1970s for RSD, this test employs a radioactive peptide which is injected into the blood and, according to the pattern of uptake, detects increased or decreased areas of bone metabolism and bone changes (e.g., patchy demineralization) in the affected limb. Some physicians may also use bone scans to monitor response to treatment. A newer bone scan, called the *triphasic bone scan* offers a higher degree of specificity for the diagnosis of RSD and is done in three stages:

  - *arteriogram* measures the uptake of the radioactive material, with increased uptake suggestive of RSD
  - *blood-pool stage* - increased activity in the joints in close proximity to the affected region is suggestive of RSD
  - *delayed stage* (3-4 hours later) - diffuse asymmetric uptake in the small joints is suggestive of RSD

- Magnetic Resonance Imaging (MRI) may be used when other imaging studies are not recommended (e.g., during pregnancy). MRI helps visualize:

  - periarticular marrow edema - swelling caused by increase of fluid around the cartilage of the affected joint
  - joint effusion - increase of fluid within the joint space
  - soft tissue swelling

Other Diagnostic Studies

Other studies that may be used in the diagnostic workup of the patient include:

Skin Temperature Measurement

The tests for skin temperature measurement track blood flow and measure the differences in temperature between the affected limb and the contralateral limb. There are three methods used to measure skin temperature:

- *Infrared Thermometry* - This test records the distribution of skin temperature in different areas of the skin of the affected limb and compares them to skin temperature on the unaffected side.

- *Laser Doppler Flowmetry* - This test measures blood flow at the level of the capillaries in response to thermal stimulation. It measures a larger area than infrared thermometry. The efficacy of Laser Doppler Flowmetry for diagnosis of RSD is a subject of debate; however, the information it provides regarding abnormalities or changes in blood perfusion is important.
- *Infrared Thermography* - This test uses an apparatus to create computer-generated images that chart changes in temperature of the affected limb. It can record changes as small as one-tenth of one degree centigrade.

Sudomotor Function Tests

Sudomotor function tests evaluate the sweat response of the affected limb. There are three tests that may be used:

- Resting Sweat Output (RSO) - this is a base measurement of sweat secretion.
- Thermoregulatory Test - this measures sweat secretion following the heating of the body. The patient is covered with an orange powder and the body is then gently heated. The orange powder turns purple where there is sweat secretion. Differences and abnormalities in the pattern of sweat production are noted.
- Quantitative Sudomotor Axon Reflex Test (QSART) - this test evaluates small nerve fibers that are linked to sweat glands. It is also effective in quantifying allodynia that is associated with RSD. Mild electrical stimulation is passed through four electrodes (three on the leg and one on the wrist) that stimulate the sweat glands and the response is measured. In addition, a tingling sensation caused by the electrical stimulus is measured subjectively (by patient report). A combination of an abnormal RSO and an abnormal QSART response results in a 98% specificity of a diagnosis of RSD. QSART, however, is not widely available.

Neurophysiological Tests

Neurophysiological tests measure nerve responses to stimulation. There are two types of tests that may be considered for RSD, including:

- *Nerve Conduction Velocity* - electrodes are placed on the skin at various locations and a mild current is passed through the electrodes. The speed at which the signal travels through the peripheral nerve is measured and any abnormalities are noted.
- *Quantitative Sensory Testing* - this test evaluates damage to small nerve endings that detect temperature changes, and to large nerve endings that detect vibration. It assesses the severity and location of nerve damage. The procedure is noninvasive. The patient feels hot and cold sensations and mild vibration. Nerve responses are then compared to the patient's unaffected side as well as to standard measurements for patients unaffected by RSD. Quantitative sensory testing is considered to be useful for confirming RSD but not for determining a diagnosis.

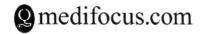

<u>*Sympathetic Nerve Blocks*</u>

Some clinicians may perform a sympathetic nerve block in order to determine if the source of the pain is sympathetically-maintained or sympathetically-independent. A local anesthetic or pain-relieving medication is injected into the sympathetic ganglion (nerve bundle). If the patient experiences pain relief following the block, it means that the pain is sympathetically-maintained and that it may respond to additional sympathetic nerve blocks or sympathectomy (surgical removal of part of a sympathetic nerve) as treatment options. Nerve blocks are not considered to be very reliable for the diagnosis of RSD because only a subset of patients with sympathetically-maintained pain respond to nerve blocks. In addition, as an invasive procedure, some clinicians are concerned about the risk-benefit ratio of causing permanent nerve damage.

Since the sympathetic nerve block can lead to complications as well as false negative or false positive results, some clinicians also perform a *phentolamine test*. Phentolamine, an antagonist for pain receptors of the sympathetic nervous system, is infused intravenously and if pain relief is achieved and is correlated to the time of infusion, it reflects involvement of the sympathetic nervous system.

In light of the fact that to date, there is no test that has been validated for the diagnosis of RSD, it is important that patients check with their health insurance companies to confirm whether any tests ordered by their doctors are covered by their health insurance policy.

Differential Diagnosis of Reflex Sympathetic Dystrophy

A variety of other conditions can mimic the signs and symptoms of reflex sympathetic dystrophy (RSD) and have to be ruled out before a definite diagnosis of RSD can be established. These include:

- Rheumatoid arthritis
- Gout
- Lumbar or cervical disk herniation
- Peripheral neuropathy, diabetic neuropathy
- Nerve entrapment syndromes (e.g., carpal tunnel syndrome)
- Osteomyelitis (bone infection)
- Septic arthritis
- Thoracic outlet syndrome
- Cellulitis
- Vascular insufficiency
- Lymphedema
- Bursitis

- Tendonitis
- Patella (kneecap) injuries
- Meniscal tears
- Femoral/tibial injury or fracture

As noted above, RSD is also known as CRPS (complex regional pain syndrome) Type I. CRPS Type II is also a cause of severe pain; however, it is due to a documented nerve injury. It is very important that a competent and experienced physician be involved in the diagnostic process since there are several aspects of CRPS Types I and II that are common to both and must be considered. These include:

- Intractable pain may be spontaneous or induced by light touch (allodynia) and exaggerated (hyperalgesia)
- Pain is not limited to the area of one specific nerve
- Pain is severe and disproportionate to the precipitating event
- There may be evidence of edema, vasomotor (blood vessel changes), and sudomotor (sweat response) abnormalities in the region of pain from the time of the precipitating event.

Guidelines for Diagnosis of Reflex Sympathetic Dystrophy

There is no consensus at this time as to how many *signs* (objective signs of dysfunction) or *symptoms* (subjective signs of dysfunction) must be present for an accurate diagnosis of reflex sympathetic dystrophy (RSD). The first formal guidelines for diagnosis of RSD were published by the International Association for the Study of Pain (IASP) in 1994 which specified four characteristic features that are required for the diagnosis of RSD. In 2006, the Reflex Sympathetic Dystrophy Syndrome Association (RSDSA) published the latest treatment guidelines for RSD that can be viewed at http://www.guideline.gov/summary/summary.aspx?ss=15&doc_id=9768&nbr=5233.

The latest criteria for the diagnosis of RSD include:

- Continuous pain that is disproportionate to the precipitating injury
- At least one symptom (reported by the patient) in three of the following four categories:
  - sensory - allodynia and/or hyperesthesia
  - vasomotor - temperature asymmetry and/or skin color changes and/or skin color asymmetry
  - sudomotor/edema - sweating changes and/or sweating asymmetry and/or

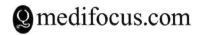

edema
- motor/trophic - decreased range of motion and/or motor dysfunction (weakness, tremor, dystonia) and/or trophic changes (hair, nail, skin)

- At least one sign (observed by clinician at the time of diagnosis) of symptoms mentioned above in two or more of the following categories:

  - sensory
  - vasomotor
  - sudomotor/edema
  - motor/trophic

- There is no other medical diagnosis that would account for the signs and symptoms

To read more about the diagnostic criteria for RSD, please click on the following link: http://www.ncbi.nlm.nih.gov/pubmed/16772794

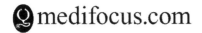
Treatment of Reflex Sympathetic Dystrophy

Goals of Treatment for Reflex Sympathetic Dystrophy

Currently, there is no cure for reflex sympathetic dystrophy (RSD) because the underlying disease process is still not well understood. Treatment, therefore, is aimed at controlling and reducing the severity of the symptoms. In general, early diagnosis and treatment is associated with a more favorable prognosis (outlook). Therapy for RSD becomes more complex and invasive as the patient's response to conventional treatments diminishes and the various aspects of the condition, especially pain, intensify. The longer the symptoms of RSD persist, the more probable it becomes that psychosocial factors will play a significant role in the patient's condition, which will then require special attention.

The goals of treatment for reflex sympathetic dystrophy include:

- Controlling and minimizing pain
- Functional rehabilitation of the affected limb
- Treatment of other existing symptoms
- Prevention of progression and worsening of RSD symptoms
- Improving the patient's quality of life and psychosocial functioning

Reflex sympathetic dystrophy has been called by some researchers a *biopsychosocial disorder*, meaning that it is a condition affecting biological, physiological, psychological, behavioral, and social aspects of the patient's life, and each of these aspects of RSD must be addressed. Thus, the treatment program for RSD requires a multidisciplinary team of medical professionals to manage all the clinical dimensions which may include:

- Primary care physician
- Neurologist
- Pain management specialist
- Surgeon
- Psychologist
- Occupational therapist
- Physical therapist
- Recreational therapist
- Vocational therapist

To read more about the efficacy of a multidisciplinary approach to pain management for RSD, please click on the following link: http://www.ncbi.nlm.nih.gov/pubmed/16868593

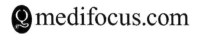

While many people suffering from RSD will benefit from intensive multidisciplinary treatment for RSD, there are others for whom the pain remains intractable and unresponsive. It is very important that these patients be taught skills in order to cope with their pain and receive counseling to try and help them improve their quality of life despite their ongoing symptoms.

Treatment Options for Reflex Sympathetic Dystrophy

Although the success of treatment for reflex sympathetic dystrophy (RSD) varies from patient to patient, there is general agreement that early-diagnosed RSD responds better to treatment than established or long-standing RSD. It is important, therefore, to start intensive treatment as soon as possible after the diagnosis of RSD has been established.

In general, the following treatment options may be considered for the management of patients with RSD:

- Functional rehabilitation
- Drug therapy
- Interventional therapy
- Psychosocial therapy

Functional Rehabilitation

Functional restoration and remobilization of the affected limb is the most important goal of therapy for reflex sympathetic dystrophy (RSD). Any other treatments, such as drug therapy or nerve blocks are employed only in order to reduce pain so that the patient can take advantage of intensive efforts to restore function. There are four components to functional rehabilitation: physical therapy, occupational therapy, recreational therapy, and vocational therapy. Treatment should begin as soon as possible after diagnosis of RSD. Restoration of function requires active participation from the patient, not passive cooperation. Patients must undertake to practice skills that they learn in various therapy settings and remain motivated to move to the next level of function under the watchful eye of the therapist even though it may cause a temporary increase in pain. It is very important for all members of the rehabilitation team to communicate, since each therapist is needed to reinforce goals set out by the others. For example, when the patient is ready to go back to work, the vocational therapist will need to inform each member of the rehabilitation team of the skills the patient needs to improve upon in order to successfully return to employment.

Each of these functional therapies involves helping the patient increase the range of motion, strength, and flexibility of the affected limb. It is important for the patient to "stay the course" and work through the difficulty of therapy since for most patients the pain will dissipate and function will return. Some of the components of functional rehabilitation include:

- Progression from gentle movements of the limb to bearing increasing weight
- Desensitization of the limb to sensory stimuli in order to "reprogram" or "reset" the way the nervous system processes this information

Additional treatments for pain control may be needed if the patient does not progress at a steady rate within a reasonable time frame. In general, professionals need to be flexible regarding when to consider the initiation of adjunct treatment because some patients derive more benefit from rehabilitation when it is accompanied by adjunct therapy early in the treatment process. Each success in rehabilitation therapy motivates the patient to continue working towards recovery, even though the process may be arduous. Therapy for coexisting conditions such as depression may need to be initiated at any stage of treatment because the patient's mental and emotional health has a significant impact on rehabilitation and recovery.

The information provided in this section is based primarily on guidelines published in the *Clinical Journal of Pain* in 2006. For further information, please click on the following link: http://www.ncbi.nlm.nih.gov/pubmed/16772795

Physical Therapy

Physical therapy (PT) is considered a cornerstone, first-line treatment for RSD and may be employed alone or in combination with other treatments such as nerve blocks and drug therapy. It should complement the other rehabilitation modalities of occupational, recreational, and vocational therapy. The primary goals of physical therapy are to:

- Restore function of the affected limb
- Alleviate pain
- Strengthen muscles in the affected limb
- Reduce swelling and joint stiffness in the affected limb

The steps to achieve these goals include:

- Helping the patient understand the importance of using the limb despite the pain. The patient and the physical therapist should set goals and a timetable of increasing demand and intensity.
- Educating the patient regarding avoidance of situations that will add stress on the

affected limb. It is important for all physical therapy to take place at the patient's level of tolerance since more aggressive therapy can trigger more pain and increase inflammation. Patients should also be counseled to avoid inactivity of the limb, prolonged bed rest, prolonged use of cold compresses, and bathing in water that is too cold.

- Raising the tolerance level for touch and desensitizing the affected area by providing sensory stimulation of increasing intensity and duration.

- Increasing functional use of the limb through:

  - increasing flexibility with range-of-motion exercises
  - increasing muscle strength with isometric exercises
  - increasing strength and flexibility through weight-bearing exercises
  - exercising on a mat which provides a non-weight-bearing setting
  - improving posture and balance (for lower extremity RSD)
  - movement training to teach proper movement patterns
  - gait training (if a leg is involved)
  - treatment for myofascial pain of proximal joints
  - aquatic therapy (hydrotherapy) in a pool or whirlpool offers the advantage of added resistance during exercise (with or without weight bearing) with less stress to the joints. The compression of water may also help if the limb is edematous (swollen). In addition, aquatic therapy is a safe way to initiate lower extremity weight-bearing and to restore functions such as walking.
  - massage therapy to manage edema and myofascial pain
  - contrast baths in warmer and cooler temperatures to help increase blood circulation to the affected limb may be efficacious for mild RSD.
  - teaching the patient to avoid "stressors" that can exacerbate pain and dysfunction in the limb, such as too little activity or too much exercise of the affected limb.

Motion exercises are important for the whole limb, not just for the joint that is affected, since the movement increases blood circulation around the joints which provides nutrition for the cartilage and decreases the hypersensitivity of the area. This prevents or minimizes contracture of the limb. Patients with advanced RSD should be treated aggressively to manage myofascial pain that occurs typically in the supporting joints of the affected limb. Some clinicians are of the opinion that if the myofascial pain can be treated successfully, other symptoms of RSD may begin to resolve.

As mentioned above, while undergoing PT, some patients benefit from drug therapy and psychotherapy so that the pain of physical therapy does not discourage them from fully cooperating and carrying out the treatment plan. Current data has shown benefit from physical therapy for the short-term, but long-term benefit has not yet been determined by clinical trials.

In children, PT combined with *Cognitive Behavioral Therapy* has been shown to provide significant improvement in measures of pain and function as well as to have a sustained benefit. Children also benefit for the long-term from aerobics, hydrotherapy and desensitization when combined with psychological counseling.

An additional treatment for RSD that may be incorporated into PT is called *mirror therapy* in which the patient sits in front of a mirror in such a way that he/she is able to see only the unaffected limb. As the patient looks in the mirror and painlessly exercises the unaffected limb (which the brain "sees" as being the affected limb due to the reverse image of the mirror), he/she can begin to move the affected limb without raising a "pain flag" from the brain. The mirror provides visual feedback for the brain so that the brain "sees" that there is no pain from the moving limb that appears to be the affected limb, leading to decreased pain and in some cases, resolution of pain. Mirror therapy is based on the theory that the cause of RSD is due to the brain "remembering" the pain from the initial injury and continually reacting with pain to any stimulation (either movement or sensory) of the limb. The therapy attempts to "re-train" the brain by "showing" it that there is no source for the pain, assuring the brain that the limb is "fine", and thereby breaking the brain's feedback loop which continually signals pain.

In a letter to the editor published in 2009 in *New England Journal of Medicine* (vol. 361(6):634-6) a study was reported that randomized 24 post-stroke patients who had developed RSD in an arm to one of three treatment groups - one that sat in front of a mirror (active-mirror group), one that sat in front of a covered mirror, and one that received training in mental imagery. The authors reported that mirror therapy effectively reduced pain and enhanced motor function not only for patients who were initially placed in the active-mirror group, but also for patients from the other groups who were later switched and received active-mirror therapy.

In another study, investigators published a review of the effectiveness of mirror therapy for upper extremity function in which they reported that mirror therapy appeared to be effective in upper limb treatment for patients with RSD and patients affected by stroke. For more information about this systematic review of mirror therapy, please click on the following link: http://www.ncbi.nlm.nih.gov/pubmed/19479545

Occupational Therapy

Occupational therapy (OT) plays a major role in the process of functional restoration. The occupational therapist will evaluate:

- Range of motion

- Edema
- Pain and abnormal sensations
- Skin changes
- Skin temperature
- Level of dexterity and muscle coordination
- Use or limitation of the affected limb in activities of daily living (ADLs)

The goals of occupational therapy for RSD include:

- Reducing or minimizing edema through the use of specialized compression garments (elasticized sleeves customized to fit the patient's arm or leg). In addition, *manual lymphatic drainage*, a gentle manual treatment technique, is designed to stimulate the flow of lymph from the congested area where it has accumulated into more centrally located lymphatic vessels that eventually return the lymph back into the venous circulation. There is also some evidence that manual lymphatic drainage may reduce pain levels as well.
- Reversing allodynia by desensitizing the skin through progressive stimulation using different textures such as feathers, silk, terrycloth, other cloth materials, and environmental textures.
- Increasing range of motion through activities such as gentle stretching, and reducing muscle "guarding" through various methods such as relaxation.
- Increasing the functional use of the limb for increased independence. Normalizing the use of the limb is strongly promoted in the rehabilitation process. This is achieved through a "stress-loading" program that involves two aspects: active movement of the limb and compression of the affected joints by increasing weight that is placed on them. For example, one activity to promote stress-loading of the upper extremity is "scrubbing", which involves back-and-forth movements using a scrub brush of increasing weight. As therapy progresses, the duration of the activity and weight applied is gradually increased.
  Another activity is "carrying" where the patient carries items of increasing weight in the hand or may apply greater weight on the foot while walking. Although stress-loading activities may initially lead to increased pain and swelling of the affected limb, after several days these symptoms usually abate.

Following edema reduction and stress-loading, OT focuses on functional restoration through exercises emphasizing range of motion, coordination, dexterity, and muscle strengthening. *Proprioceptive neuromuscular facilitation* is an advanced form of flexibility training that includes systematic stretching and contraction of targeted muscle groups.

Recreational Therapy

Because recreational therapists (RT) promote leisure activities that are pleasurable, they are often effective in motivating patients to work hard in rehabilitation. "Fun" activities can also be instrumental in helping the patient overcome fear of using the affected limb *(kinesphobia)*. While focusing on the enjoyable activity, such as videogames, the patient "forgets" the fear and begins to use the limb. By coordinating with the occupational therapist and physical therapist, the recreational therapist can choose activities that augment the goals set for the patient.

Another role the recreational therapist plays in the rehabilitation of patients with RSD is helping them become more involved in social and community activities. By practicing skills needed for activities patients enjoy doing with friends or family, the recreational therapist helps motivate patients to participate actively in their recovery. The recreational therapist also helps patients to get involved in activities they once enjoyed or would like to learn, such as gardening, bowling, and dancing. Patients may start out by using modified equipment such as large-handled utensils or light-weight bowling balls in order to build up motivation and success in carrying out activities. Leisure skills, recreational activities, and increased participation in social opportunities promote self-confidence in patients and reduce fear of using the affected limb.

Vocational Therapy

Vocational therapy (VT) is an important step in the rehabilitation process since it impacts strongly on the patient's health status, quality of life, and self-image. It is often the last stage of therapy and serves to prepare patients for return to the workplace - either to their former job or to a new job which will fit their skill level. This step is also important since relapse seems to be more likely when a person is inactive.

The role of the vocational therapist includes:

- Determining if patients can successfully go back to their former place of employment, or planning skills that the patient should be working on to prepare for returning to their former workplace
- Determining if the work environment needs to be modified for the level of the patient's skills
- Visiting the work-site and coordinating the patient's needs with the needs of the employer. The therapist may initiate a trial period for the patient to return to work under observation so that any issues that may need to be addressed (such as the increased need for rest breaks or a modified work schedule) may be addressed.
- Helping patients navigate issues that may arise with their return to employment such as health insurance changes, or any legal issues that may be related to patients' disabilities.
- Investigating new employment opportunities that would be appropriate for patients who cannot return to their former workplace.
- Explaining the steps patients may need to take to collect disability insurance, health insurance, and other governmental or legal claims which may need to be filed.

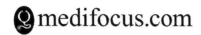
The vocational therapist may see the patient after they have been unemployed for an extended period of time due to RSD by which point the patient's self image, motivation to work, and motivation to recover may have suffered significantly. While coordinating with the physical therapist and occupational therapist, the vocational therapist can help patients set realistic expectations regarding their opportunities for employment and can help them focus on acquiring the skills that will be needed in the workplace.

Drug Therapy for Reflex Sympathetic Dystrophy

Prompt initiation of medications for reflex sympathetic dystrophy (RSD) is very important, especially if the pain is intense, in order to enable the patient to proceed with therapy necessary for functional restoration. During the course of treatment, medication doses may have to be adjusted to achieve optimal pain relief and to facilitate the patient's cooperation and participation in physical and occupational therapy. There is a shortage of information regarding effective pharmacotherapy for RSD due to limited numbers of randomized controlled trials. Most medications are prescribed based either on anecdotal evidence (patients have reported that a particular medication was effective for them) or based on studies that have shown that particular medications are effective for other neuropathic pain conditions such as peripheral neuropathy or trigeminal neuralgia.

There are no guidelines regarding a first-line medication for RSD. As a result, there is typically an initial trial-and-error period until the most effective medication is found. At that point, there may be a period of several adjustments until the correct dose is determined. Direct comparisons of the efficacy of drug therapy vs. other therapies such as physical therapy alone, nerve blocks, or spinal stimulation have not yet been investigated.

The 2006 Clinical Guidelines for Treatment of RSD published by the Reflex Sympathetic Dystrophy Syndrome Association (RSDSA) note that in most cases, no single drug will be sufficient to manage symptoms over the long-term, and that two or more medications will be needed to manage RSD-associated pain. For this reason, it is important for physicians treating RSD to be intimately aware of interactions between drugs used for treatment of RSD both in terms of those that are complementary when given together and those that may be contraindicated as simultaneous therapies.

There are various classes of drugs that may be used for the treatment of RSD including:

- Analgesics
- Anticonvulsants
- Antidepressants
- Bisphosphonates

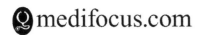

- Muscle relaxants
- Adrenergic active drugs
- Steroids
- Opioids

Analgesics (Pain Medications)

- Aspirin
- Acetaminophen
- Non-steroidal anti-inflammatory drugs (NSAIDs)

Side effects include:

- Nausea/vomiting
- Diarrhea
- Constipation
- Thinning of the blood (aspirin)

Anticonvulsants

A variety of anticonvulsants have been used in RSD patients to provide pain relief including:

- Gabapentin (Neurontin) - this is part of a class of drugs called *GABA (gamma-aminobutyric acid) analogues* that increase the availability of GABA in the blood resulting in a relaxing, anti-anxiety, or anti-convulsant effect. Gabapentin has been proven to be effective in clinical trials for neuropathic pain. Although there are no clinical trials showing efficacy for RSD, there is sufficient anecdotal evidence for pain relief that gabapentin is recommended by clinicians for treatment of RSD. Gabapentin does not appear to improve functional impairment.
- Pregabalin (Lyrica) - this drug is also a GABA-analogue. It was approved by the U.S. Food and Drug Administration (FDA) in 2004 for neuropathic pain of diabetic neuropathy, and in 2007 for treatment of fibromyalgia. Some physicians use pregabalin "off label" (to treat conditions other than those approved by the FDA for a particular medication) for the management of RSD pain. To date, no randomized trials have been conducted to evaluate the efficacy of pregabalin for treatment of RSD.
- Carbamazepine (Tegretol)
- Phenytoin (Dilantin)

Side effects of anticonvulsants include:

- Dizziness

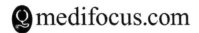
- Drowsiness
- Nausea/vomiting
- Abnormalities of blood or platelet counts
- Abnormalities of liver function

Anticonvulsant Medications and Suicidality

In August 2009, the U.S. Food and Drug Administration (FDA) issued an alert for healthcare professionals that the labeling of anticonvulsant (anti-seizure) drugs will now warn that patients taking these drugs have an increased risk of suicidal thoughts and actions. The warnings are based on FDA's analysis of placebo-controlled clinical studies of eleven drugs used to treat epilepsy, psychiatric disorders, and other conditions. In this analysis, the risk of suicidal thoughts and actions was almost doubled in patients taking the anticonvulsant medications compared with those receiving a placebo (0.43% vs. 0.22%).

The following anticonvulsant drugs were included in the FDA's analysis:

- Carbamazepine (Carbatrol; Equetro; Tegretol)
- Felbamate (Felbatol)
- Gabapentin (Neurontin)
- Lamotrigine (Lamictal)
- Levetiracetam (Keppra)
- Oxcarbazepine (Trileptal)
- Pregabalin (Lyrica)
- Tiagabine (Gabitril)
- Topiramate (Topamax)
- Valproate (Depakote; Depakene; Depacon)
- Zonisamide (Zonegran)

The increased risk of suicidal thoughts and actions was observed as early as one-week after starting therapy with these anticonvulsant drugs and continued through 24 weeks. The increased risk was generally consistent for all eleven drugs included in the analysis and across a range of indications. This suggests that this risk applies to all anticonvulsant medications when they are used for any indication - even those drugs that were not part of the analysis.

The FDA urges healthcare professionals to monitor closely all patients starting or taking anticonvulsant medications. They should be alert to changes in behavior that could signal an emerging or worsening of depression or suicidal thoughts and behavior. Patients will also be provided with Medication Guides explaining these risks each time their anticonvulsant medication prescriptions are dispensed.

Antidepressants

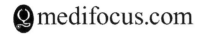

There are three types of antidepressants that may be considered in the treatment of RSD:

- *Tricyclic antidepressants* (TCAs) may be very effective for RSD based on anecdotal evidence; however, they carry a risk of intentional overdose which may result in death. There is also considerable concern regarding the anticholinergic side-effects (such as confusion, blurred vision, or light-headedness) and cardiac side-effects (such as increased heart rate or low blood pressure) especially in patients with a history of prior heart disease). Tricyclic antidepressants that may be used in the treatment of RSD include:

  - amitriptyline (Elavil)
  - doxepin (Sinequan, Adapin)
  - nortriptyline (Pamelor, Aventyl)

- *Selective serotonin reuptake inhibitors* (SSRIs) are not as prone to overdose; however, they are also not as effective for the treatment of pain in RSD. Selective serotonin reuptake inhibitors that may be effective for treatment of RSD include:

  - fluoxetine (Prozac)
  - sertraline (Zoloft)
  - paroxetine (Paxil)

- *Selective serotonin and norepinephrine reuptake inhibitors* (SNRIs) have been shown to be effective in relieving chronic neuropathic pain and may be effective for RSD as well. These include:

  - venlafaxine (Effexor)
  - duloxetine (Cymbalta)

Some clinicians suggest that SSRIs should be used for patients who have failed to find relief from TCAs or SNRIs. In general, although antidepressants may be effective for some patients with RSD, none have been approved by the FDA for the treatment of RSD.

Side effects of antidepressants include:

- Nausea/vomiting
- Dry mouth
- Urine retention
- Sleep disruption
- Weight gain
- Anxiety

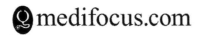

Bisphosphonates

Bisphosphonates target bone loss and have been studied more thoroughly than any other drugs for the treatment of RSD. Bisphosphonates that have undergone clinical trials for treatment of RSD include:

- Calcitonin (intranasal spray)
- Clodronate (intravenous)
- Alendronate (intravenous)

Although some clinical trials showed improvement in active movement and motor function, there are some studies where the data regarding efficacy for pain and functional improvement of RSD were inconclusive.

Side effects of bisphosphonates include:

- Fever and flu-like symptoms
- Hypocalcemia (low levels of calcium)
- Bone and joint pain - the FDA notes that some people taking bisphosphonates may experience severe and sometimes incapacitating bone, joint, and/or muscle (musculoskeletal) pain
- Kidney damage
- Osteonecrosis (breakdown of bone tissue) of the jaw
- Constipation or diarrhea

Muscle Relaxants

Muscle relaxants are used to provide relief from muscle cramps and to control muscle spasms that may be associated with RSD. Examples of muscle relaxants include:

- Clonazepam (Klonopin)
- Baclofen (Lioresal)

Side-effects of muscle relaxants include:

- Drowsiness
- Dry mouth
- Dizziness
- Fatigue
- Nausea
- Unpleasant taste in the mouth
- Blurred vision

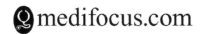

Adrenergic Agonist Drugs

Adrenergic-agonist drugs decrease the activity of the sympathetic nervous system in general and also relax certain muscles. They belong to a class of drugs known as *sympatholytic agents*. Based on anecdotal evidence, many physicians use these drugs to treat RSD-related pain, including:

- Clonidine (Catapres) - oral or transdermal patch
- Phenoxybenzamine (Dibenzyline)
- Reserpine (Harmonyl)

Studies have reported that intravenous phentolamine (Regitine) is not effective in controlling pain in RSD.

Although the mechanism of action is not entirely understood, it is thought that these adrenergic active drugs work by blocking the action of norepinephrine on nerve receptors that become active in neuropathic pain.

Side effects include:

- Nervousness
- Agitation
- Sleep disturbances

Corticosteroids

This class of drugs is used to reduce inflammation and swelling and has been used to control many types of pain for many years. After going through a period of not being used for RSD, they are once again being investigated in clinical trials for treatment of RSD-related pain. So far, corticosteroids such as prednisone and methylprednisolone have demonstrated good analgesic efficacy for patients with early-stage RSD where there are prominent symptoms and signs of inflammation. Patients must be monitored carefully for potentially serious side effects including susceptibility to infections and avascular necrosis of bone (death of bone tissue due to an inadequate blood supply).

Other side effects include:

- Weight gain
- Fluid retention
- Increased appetite
- Nervousness
- Indigestion

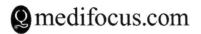

- Dizziness
- Mood swings
- Elevated pressure in the eyes (glaucoma)

When taken over a long period of time, corticosteroids can lead to cataracts and diabetes.

Oral Opioids

This class of drugs may help relieve severe cases of RSD with widespread pain. Use of opioids for RSD is controversial, although it remains the gold standard of treatment for acute pain in general. The potential side effects, however, such as drug tolerance, addiction, and drowsiness are serious considerations. Other side effects of opioids may include constipation, sedation, and dry mouth.

Opioids that may be used to treat pain in RSD include:

- Oxycodone (Oxycontin)
- Morphine
- Methadone

Tramadol (Ultram) is an *atypical opioid* that is effective for chronic neuropathic pain and may be effective for RSD as well. It is not a *controlled substance*, like other opioids such as morphine, and also has less of an effect on the gastrointestinal tract (constipation, nausea) than classic opioids.

N-Methyl-D-Aspartate (NMDA) Antagonist

Ketamine is a potent NMDA which has been studied for the treatment of RSD. Ketamine infusion therapy has been shown to be effective in acute and overall pain relief that continues beyond the duration of the infusion; however functional improvement is limited. A study published in October 2009 in *Pain* (vol. 145(3):304-1) reported that a multiple-day ketamine infusion resulted in significant pain relief in a group of patients diagnosed with RSD but there was no functional improvement of the limb.
For more information about this study, please click on the following links:
http://www.ncbi.nlm.nih.gov/pubmed/19604642

In general, medication for RSD is determined by prominent symptoms displayed by each patient. One medication may not provide sufficient relief, requiring the addition of another drug or switching to a different class of drugs. The Guidelines published by the RSDSA recommend the following medications for relief of specific symptoms:

- Mild-to-moderate pain - simple analgesics and/or blocks (see below)
- Severe, intractable pain - opioids and/or blocks or experimental interventions

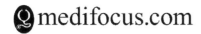

- Inflammation and edema - steroids and/or non steroidal anti-inflammatory drugs (NSAIDs)
- Depression, anxiety, insomnia - sedative, analgesic antidepressant and/or psychotherapy
- Significant allodynia - anticonvulsants and/or sodium channel blockers and/or NMDA-receptor agonists
- Significant osteopenia and trophic changes - calcitonin or bisphosphonates
- Profound vasomotor disturbance - calcium channel blockers, sympatholytics, and/or blocks

For more information about medications that are used for RSD-related pain, please click on the following link: http://www.ncbi.nlm.nih.gov/pubmed/20054678

Interventional Procedures for Reflex Sympathetic Dystrophy

Interventional therapies have been commonly used in the treatment of reflex sympathetic dystrophy (RSD) even without scientific evidence of their efficacy. The basic premise of most interventional treatments was the involvement of the sympathetic nervous system in RSD, a premise which has come under increasing scrutiny in the face of new evidence of more systemic involvement.

The role of interventional treatment in RSD is that of an adjunct therapy performed in order to provide pain relief to enable patients to participate actively in functional rehabilitation. The decision to undergo interventional therapy should be considered carefully regarding the level of need, timing, and whether it will be more effective for pain relief than other therapies which may have been undertaken and failed.

Interventional procedures include:

- Nerve block
- Sympathectomy
- Spinal Cord/Peripheral Nerve Stimulation
- Implantable Spinal Pumps

You can read more about various interventional procedures for treatment of RSD by clicking on the following link: http://www.ncbi.nlm.nih.gov/pubmed/19300041

Nerve Block
A nerve block is a procedure usually performed by a pain management specialist (anesthesiologist) and its objective is to interrupt the flow of pain signals along the

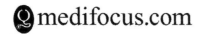

sympathetic nerve in the region of RSD pain. If successful, the anesthetic temporarily blocks the local sympathetic nervous system and thus reduces or eliminates pain.

Based on clinical experience, some doctors recommend a nerve block in the presence of any of the following conditions:

- Burning pain
- Allodynia
- Temperature changes in the affected limb
- Color changes in the affected limb
- Limited success with functional rehabilitation despite medication

There are three types of nerve blocks. Two target the sympathetic nervous system, and one that targets local nerves in the affected limb. The procedures that target the sympathetic nervous system include:

- *Stellate ganglion block* - Anesthetic is injected around the sympathetic nerves in the cervical spine to interrupt pain signals to the upper body and arm.

- *Lumbar sympathetic block* - Anesthetic is injected around the sympathetic nerves in the lumbar region and targets interruption of nerve signals causing lower body/leg pain.

Until recently, sympathetic nerve block played an important role in the diagnosis and treatment of RSD. If a sympathetic nerve block was performed on a patient and there was relief from pain, the diagnosis of RSD was confirmed. Currently, however, since there is ongoing debate over the exclusive role of the sympathetic nervous system in RSD, nerve block plays a less prominent role, although it is still performed often. There are few rigorous studies on any of these nerve blocks in RSD and data is unclear regarding long-term efficacy.

If the sympathetic nerve block is effective, it usually provides immediate, although temporary, pain relief and also increases the patient's level of comfort and function. This provides the patient with a window of opportunity for more intense efforts to restore function with increased physical therapy. In addition, this procedure does not interfere with motor activity so the patient can remain mobile and active after nerve block administration. Recurrence of pain after the initial nerve block occurs in many patients and subsequent sympathetic nerve blocks or stronger measures are required.

Despite popular opinion, there is little evidence-based information regarding the best timing for administering nerve blocks, how many times it should be administered, or its long-term efficacy. In any event, nerve blockade should always be accompanied by aggressive physical rehabilitation. Because a variety of complications can occur following a nerve block, it is prudent for patients to select a pain management specialist, such as an anesthesiologist, who is experienced with this technique.

Potential complications that may result from sympathetic nerve blocks include:

- Nerve injury
- Bleeding - nerve blocks are usually contraindicated in patients who are taking anticoagulant medications
- Allergic reactions to local anesthetics
- Psychological reactions - anxiety and fear related to apprehension about the nerve block procedure
- Cardiac arrest (reported with lidocaine and bupivacaine only)
- Seizures
- Compartment syndrome - the compression of nerves, blood vessels and muscle inside a closed space that leads to muscle and nerve damage and blood flow problems

There are no universally accepted guidelines regarding the choice of anesthetic for the blockade, which patients benefit the most from the blockade, and which type of nerve block is most effective. The most commonly used anesthetic is lidocaine.

The third type of nerve block targets nerves in the affected limb and is called a *Bier block* or *Intravenous Regional Anesthesia* block (IVRA). With this procedure, blood is drained from the limb either by gravity (holding the limb up) or pressure. A blood pressure cuff is then inflated at the upper arm or leg and an anesthetic is injected intravenously into a blood vessel in the hand or foot. The inflated cuff prevents the anesthetic from flowing out of the limb and into the body. The patient may feel a burning sensation and numbness as the anesthetic diffuses from the blood vessels into nearby nerves. The procedure ends by slowly deflating the pressure cuff, allowing the small amount of residual anesthetic to slowly flow out of the limb through the veins into the body where it is resorbed. The numbness eventually wears off. Pain relief is temporary and may last days, weeks, or months. When the effect wears off, the procedure can be repeated. The main complication of the Bier block is that if the pressure cuff is released too quickly, before a sufficient amount of anesthetic has been absorbed into the arm, too much anesthetic is introduced into the body and can reach toxic levels.

Surgery and IVRA

Evidence shows patients with RSD of the upper extremity benefit when IVRA is performed prior to undergoing surgery of the affected limb. A study was published in which 84 patients with a history of RSD were to undergo surgery of the affected upper

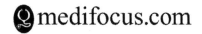

extremity. All of the patients received an infusion of lidocaine combined with either clonidine or saline (control group). The RSD recurrence rate of the group receiving lidocaine and clonidine was significantly lower than the group receiving lidocaine and saline (10% vs. 74%).

Sympathectomy

Sympathectomy is a procedure that is intended to destroy the collection of sympathetic nerve cells (*sympathetic ganglion*) along the spinal cord and to suppress or block the sympathetically-maintained pain in the affected area. Because a sympathectomy is a procedure that carries significant risks (which will be discussed below) and the outcome may vary from patient to patient, the decision to undergo this procedure should be carefully assessed. Patients who are offered a surgical sympathectomy as a treatment option should carefully investigate the surgeon's experience and success rate with this procedure before making the decision to proceed with it.

Patients are considered as potential candidates for sympathectomy only if response to a sympathetic nerve block shows that the source of the RSD pain is sympathetically-maintained pain. If the source of the RSD pain is determined to be sympathetically-independent pain (i.e., no reduction of pain is noted after a nerve block), a sympathectomy is not a viable treatment option.

There are 2 types of sympathectomy:

- Chemical sympathectomy
- Surgical sympathectomy

Chemical Sympathectomy

During a chemical sympathectomy, a *neurolytic agent* (a chemical that destroys nerve cells) is injected into the sympathetic ganglion at a specific site to block sympathetically-maintained pain. Phenol and ethanol are the two most frequently used neurolytic agents for chemical sympathectomy. Chemical sympathectomy typically provides temporary relief and only for patients with cutaneous allodynia (abnormal sensitivity to touch). One study published in 2001 in *Clinical Journal of Pain* (vol. 17:327-336) reported that efficacy of chemical sympathectomy performed on 66 patients with RSD was as follows:

- 44% experienced meaningful relief
- 19% reported no relief
- 37% reached no conclusion due to poor reporting of outcome in the study

Potential complications of chemical sympathectomy include:

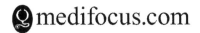

- Post-sympathectomy pain
- Paralysis
- Neuritis - inflammation of a nerve due to irritation from the phenol or ethanol

Surgical Sympathectomy

A surgical sympathectomy involves cutting and cauterizing (sealing) the nerves of the sympathetic ganglion at a specific location along the spinal cord. There are various techniques that may be used to perform a surgical sympathectomy, including *video-assisted surgery*, *open surgery*, or *radiofrequency sympathectomy* (use of a heated electrode to destroy the nerves).

Following a surgical sympathectomy, the patient may experience complete pain relief, partial pain relief, or no pain relief. In general, many patients experience complete or partial pain relief for several months following a surgical sympathectomy but only about 15% to 30% experience long-term relief lasting two years or longer.

In a study published in 2002 in the *Journal of Vascular Surgery*, researchers from the University of South Florida College of Medicine reported that approximately 90% of patients with RSD in their study who underwent surgical sympathectomy reported at least a 50% reduction in pain intensity, although the level of pain reduction deteriorated over time. Ten percent of the patients in this study were considered treatment failures. A significant subset of the total patients regretted having undergone the procedure due to subsequent reported high levels of disability. Overall patient satisfaction was 77%.

You can read more about this study by clicking on the following link:
http://www.ncbi.nlm.nih.gov/pubmed/11854724

Potential complications of surgical sympathectomy include:

- Post-sympathectomy pain - reported to occur in about 40% of patients
- Compensatory hyperhidrosis - excessive sweating of the face, trunk, or legs
- Recurrence of RSD pain
- Pneumothorax - accidental injury to the lung (for upper body RSD)
- Horner's syndrome - injury to the sympathetic nerves of the face which includes a constricted pupil, drooping eyelids, and facial dryness
- Postural hypotension - a drop in blood pressure due to a change in body position (such as from a sitting to standing position)

A review of sympathectomy as a treatment for neuropathic pain was published in the *Cochrane Database of Systematic Reviews* in 2003. The reviewers concluded that the evidence regarding the efficacy of sympathectomy is based on "poor quality evidence, uncontrolled study, and personal experience". In addition, there may be significant

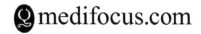

complications including worsening of pain, development of a new pain syndrome, and abnormal patterns of sweating. To read more about this review of sympathectomy, please click on the following link: http://www.ncbi.nlm.nih.gov/pubmed/12804444

An update of the 2003 Cochrane review of sympathectomy for treatment of pain in RSD was published in 2010. The authors concluded that there was little high quality evidence of benefit of surgical or chemical sympathectomy on pain relief in individuals with RSD and they advised that it be considered only after failure of other treatment options. For more information about this updated review on sympathectomy for the treatment of RSD, please click on the following link: http://www.ncbi.nlm.nih.gov/pubmed/20614432

Generally, there is ongoing debate about this procedure in the medical community for several reasons, including:

- Significant complications
- Procedure does not sufficiently enhance the effectiveness of physical or occupational therapy
- Lack of well designed, randomized, controlled clinical trials proving efficacy of this procedure
- Debate about the key role of the sympathetic nervous system in RSD

Spinal Cord Stimulation

Another treatment option for patients with RSD is the use of electrical nerve stimulators that apply a small amount of electrical current to the nerves in the spinal cord to overcome the sensation of pain. This type of treatment is known as *spinal cord stimulation* (SCS). Since being introduced in the 1960s, spinal cord stimulation fell out of favor, but with recent advances in technology, it is being re-evaluated for its efficacy in treating chronic pain.

A spinal cord stimulator is a device that consists of a power source, wires, and an external controller. A small wire, called a *lead*, is surgically implanted into the epidural space of the spinal column and is connected to a power source implanted in the patient and an external unit controlled by the patient. When the patient initiates the flow of electrical current from the external unit, low-level electrical impulses are transmitted from the power source through the lead wire to the spinal cord to interrupt and block pain signal. Spinal cord stimulation affects the entire central nervous system. *Peripheral nerve stimulators* (PNS) are similar to spinal cord stimulators with the difference being that the electrodes are placed outside the central nervous system to target only the peripheral nerves.

In most cases, before a spinal cord stimulator is implanted permanently, a temporary stimulator is implanted for a trial period of several days to determine if the patient will experience a reduction in the level of pain. If good pain control is achieved during the trial

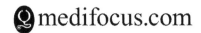
period, the next step is the surgical implantation of a permanent spinal cord stimulator. Patients with implanted device often describe the sensation of the electrical current from the SCS as a "tingling" feeling; however, these sensations are far less bothersome than the pain associated with RSD.

Spinal cord stimulators enable patients suffering from chronic RSD pain a means of better controlling their pain. Patients are usually able to resume their normal activities both at home and at work and also to participate in recreational activities, since the unit is portable. Although SCS is not a cure for chronic RSD pain, in many cases it can reduce the level of intensity of the pain and make it more manageable.

There is no consensus regarding the timing of the initiation of SCS in the rehabilitation process of RSD. In general, SCS is increasingly being considered at early stages of therapy for some cases of RSD if it will help with advancing rehabilitation. It cannot be argued that the patient should have tried all conservative therapies before considering SCS and patients should not have to wait as long as previously thought before being offered SCS as an option. In short, SCS should no longer be considered a last-resort treatment modality.

For more information about the report of this expert panel, please click on the following link: http://www.ncbi.nlm.nih.gov/pubmed/17134466

Studies indicate that many patients who undergo this procedure report a 50-70% reduction in pain, or at least enough to become functional at work or to lead an active life. A study published in the *European Journal of Pain* in February 2010 (vol. 14(2):164-9) noted that SCS fails to result in significant pain relief for one-third of RSD patients, and causes complications in 32-38% of patients who undergo the treatment. A meta-analysis that was completed in the United Kingdom was published in 2006 in *Journal of Pain and Symptom Management* (vol. 31(4 Suppl):S13-9) and reported that there is "Grade A evidence" of the efficacy of spinal cord stimulation for RSD and SCS treatment results in reducing pain, improving quality of life, enabling some patients to return to work, and reducing the amount of medication taken by some patients.

To read more about this interesting finding, please click on the following link: http://www.ncbi.nlm.nih.gov/pubmed/16647590

Though some patients report successful control of pain in studies involving SCS compared to placebo groups, there is currently no absolute proof of efficacy. There is some indication that SCS may be effective in patients who have already undergone surgical sympathectomy. In addition, there are indications that a patient's positive response to a prior sympathetic nerve block may predict a good response to SCS. Spinal cord stimulation seems to produce analgesia without any reduction of sympathetic function.

Data is limited but there is evidence of efficacy of spinal cord stimulation. In 2000, a study was published in the *New England Journal of Medicine* (vol. 343(9):618-24) and reported that a group of patients with RSD who had been treated with SCS and physical therapy experienced significant reduction of pain and increased quality of life compared to a group that was given physical therapy alone. Functional outcome in terms of day-to-day use of the affected limb, however, was no better than that experienced by the group who had received physical therapy alone.

More recently, a five-year follow-up of patients who underwent SCS was published in *Journal of Neurosurgery* and the conclusion drawn was that despite the fact that pain relief diminished over time, 95% of the patients reported that they would repeat the procedure if they could achieve the same result. For more information about this article, please click on the following link: http://www.ncbi.nlm.nih.gov/pubmed/18240925

Patients with RSD who may be considered as candidates for SCS include:

- Patients not making significant progress in rehabilitation with conservative therapy who will be able to exercise more effectively and participate in a more intensive rehabilitation protocol with increased control over pain
- Patients who are psychologically stable and have realistic expectations regarding further treatment and prognosis
- Patients who have had a favorable response to sympathetic nerve blocks but need more intense pain relief

If the patient is deemed a candidate for SCS, it is important to perform the procedure in a timely manner since waiting too long may diminish the success of the treatment.

Potential risks and complications associated with surgical implantation of the spinal cord stimulator include:

- Infection
- Headache
- Bleeding
- Spinal cord injury
- Failure to relieve pain
- Pain at the site of the implant
- Hardware malfunction

Contraindications to the use of SCS include:

- Patients with implantable devices such as a pacemaker or defibrillator
- Patients undergoing radiation therapy

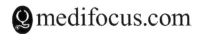
- Patients who are exposed to detection equipment devices including anti-theft devices, security devices, and aircraft communication systems

Patients who have an implanted SCS device should not drive or operate heavy equipment while the device is activated. They should also carry special identification papers through security systems (such as airports), since the system can activate metal detectors.

Spinal cord stimulation has been approved by the US Food and Drug Administration (FDA) as a treatment for RSD. The FDA approved the ANS Renew and the Medtronics Mattrix systems for SCS delivery.

Implantable Spinal Pumps

Implantable spinal pumps provide a way of delivering drugs *intrathecally*, directly into the cerebrospinal fluid. Medications are delivered within the intrathecal space (the space surrounding the spinal cord) either by injection through a needle or via a catheter that is connected to a pump. Doses can be programmed to be delivered continuously at a particular rate that can be increased or decreased, or on a schedule controlled by the patient. Medications can be opioid or non-opioid but morphine is the "gold standard" drug used in the implantable spinal pump. If the patient cannot tolerate morphine, other drugs such as baclofen or ziconotide may be tried. Long-term experience with the morphine pump in patients with chronic pain, including those with RSD, indicates few advantages over oral morphine administration. In fact, many patients with implantable morphine pumps also require oral morphine supplementation to control their pain. The implantation of a morphine pump is also associated with potential complications including:

- Infection
- Bleeding
- Spinal fluid leakage
- Injury to the spinal cord
- Malfunction of the pump

Side effects of morphine include:

- Nausea/vomiting
- Urine retention
- Itching
- Constipation
- Confusion
- Sexual dysfunction

Implantable spinal pumps are considered a last-resort therapy and should be only considered if the patient does not respond to spinal cord stimulation and/or does not have

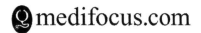

multiple pain sites. Before a patient can be considered for intrathecal medication, it is important to evaluate several factors including:

- If the patient has had any adverse response to any systemic medications
- If the patient is motivated to pursue functional rehabilitation after experiencing symptom relief from the implantable pump
- If the patient is psychologically stable and can self-control medications in an appropriate manner
- If the patient understands the risks and benefits of this therapy
- How the patient has responded to all previous treatments

Implantable spinal pump is contraindicated in the following conditions:

- If the patient is intolerant to the medications used in the pump
- If the patient has an infection
- If the patient has problems with blood clotting

Intrathecal Ziconotide

Ziconotide is a non-opioid analgesic medication that is used strictly for the management of patients with chronic, severe pain. In December 2004, the U.S. Food and Drug Administration (FDA) approved ziconotide for administration as an infusion into the cerebrospinal fluid using an intrathecal pump system. Ziconotide is a selective calcium channel blocker and provides pain relief by blocking the release of specific chemicals in the brain and spinal cord that promote the sensation of pain. Although the safety and efficacy of ziconotide have been previously demonstrated for several types of chronic pain conditions, to date there have not been many trials investigating ziconotide for treatment of RSD.

In a study published in 2009 in *Pain Practice* (Volume 9; Issue 4, pp. 296-303), researchers from the Cleveland Clinic Foundation evaluated the safety and efficacy of intrathecal ziconotide in seven patients with CRPS. Six patients included in this study had CRPS Type I (RSD) while one patient had CRPS Type II. The mean duration of CRPS among these seven patients was about 3.5 years and the mean age was 32 years. All of the patients included in this study had failed to improve with other prior treatment modalities and were considered as having CRPS that was highly refractory to treatment.

Treatment consisted of continuous infusion of intrathecal ziconotide with an implantable pump and was continued for an average of three years. The primary measure of the effectiveness of intrathecal ziconotide therapy was the percentage reduction in the level of pain from before to after treatment with ziconotide. The severity of pain was evaluated using a *visual analog scale* (VAS) ranging from a score of "0" (no pain) to "100" (worst pain imaginable). (A visual analog scale is a measurement instrument for subjective

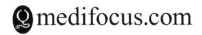

characteristics that cannot be directly measured such as pain intensity.)

The researchers reported the following major findings of their study:

- Treatment with intrathecal ziconotide resulted in a significant reduction in pain intensity as measured on VAS:

    - mean VAS pain score was 89 at the initiation of ziconotide therapy and had dropped to a mean of 43 after treatment had been completed
    - mean improvement in the VAS pain score from before to after ziconotide treatment was 51%

- Three of the seven patients included in this study had additional CRPS-related symptoms such as edema (swelling) and discoloration of the skin. Ziconotide therapy resulted in improvement of these symptoms in all three patients.

- Six of the seven patients experienced adverse side-effects from ziconotide, most of which were neuropsychiatric or cognitive in nature. These side-effects were managed by either lowering the dose of ziconotide or by temporarily discontinuing the medication.

Common side-effects of ziconotide therapy that have been reported in previous studies include:

- Dizziness
- Nausea
- Confusion
- Headache
- Weakness
- Hypertonia (increased muscle tone resulting in a reduced ability to stretch the affected muscle)
- Ataxia (unsteady movement and a staggering gait)
- Vision disturbances
- Anorexia
- Sleepiness
- Memory impairment

Severe, but rare, side-effects of ziconotide therapy that have been documented previously included:

- Hallucinations
- Suicidal thoughts

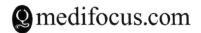
- New-onset depression or worsening of pre-existing depression
- Meningitis
- Seizures

Ziconotide is contraindicated in people with a history of psychiatric illness such as depression, psychosis, schizophrenia, and bipolar disorder.

In conclusion, the results of this study have shown that intrathecal ziconotide may be useful for the treatment of select patients with CRPS that is highly refractory to other treatment modalities. Ziconotide therapy resulted in significant improvements of other severe CRPS-related symptoms, including pain, swelling and skin discoloration. Moreover, patients treated with ziconotide showed increased levels of activity as compared to before ziconotide therapy. Although additional studies are necessary to confirm the findings of this study, nevertheless, based on the data obtained with a small number of patients, ziconotide appears to be a promising new treatment option for patients with CRPS that cannot be well-controlled with other treatment modalities.

The 2006 guidelines of the RSDSA divide interventional therapies into three groups:

- Minimally invasive therapies: Sympathetic Nerve Blocks, Intravenous Regional Nerve Blocks (IVRA), and Somatic Nerve Blocks (along various segments of the spinal cord)
- More invasive therapies: Epidural Catheter Nerve Blocks, Neurostimulation, and Intrathecal Infusion
- Surgical and experimental therapies: Sympathectomy and Motor Cortex Stimulation

Psychological Management of Reflex Sympathetic Dystrophy

While some patients with RSD may heal spontaneously within the first six to eight weeks of developing RSD or respond quickly to therapy so that they do not need to focus as intently on psychological intervention, others who do not respond quickly may develop harmful habits such as disuse of the arm or bracing the arm to protect it from injury or pain. The consensus statement of 2003 issued by the International Association for the Study of Pain recommends that psychological intervention be initiated for patients with reflex sympathetic dystrophy (RSD) experiencing pain for more than two months. Behavioral treatments may be used in the management of RSD to gain control over the pain by various methods which may enable the patient to reduce muscle spasms, pain, and improve sleep disturbances. Patients experiencing pain for longer than six months may require additional interventions.

The objectives of psychological treatment of the patient with RSD include:

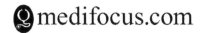
- Helping the patient overcome learned disuse of the affected limb due to fear of pain or fear of injuring the limb
- Providing coping skills for living with pain
- Introducing ways to improve quality of life despite the presence of chronic pain

Individual psychological counseling and group therapy are reported by many patients to have a positive role in therapeutic outcome for RSD as it helps them learn to manage their condition. An important aspect of treatment besides learning to live with pain is establishing functional goals in order to maintain maximum independence. Counseling also helps patients cope with their self-perception as handicapped and/or disabled people and enables them to work on maximizing their functionality.

Psychological intervention has become more recognized recently as an integral part of management of RSD and is included in the 2006 Guidelines of Diagnosis and Treatment for RSD published by the Reflex Sympathetic Dystrophy Syndrome Association (RSDSA).

The RSDSA Guidelines recommend that psychological management include three parts:

- Education of the patient and family
- Psychological assessment
- Pain management skills

Education of Patient and Family

Educating the patient and family about RSD should be initiated as soon as medical/rehabilitation therapy begins, regarding issues such as:

- Negative effect of disuse and neglect of the affected extremity
- Importance of using the extremity in order to regain function
- Understanding the relationship between behaviors to protect the limb from pain and the ongoing severity of RSD.
- Understanding that patients must be active participants in therapy which involves: being ready to work through the increase of pain that may occur when each new level of therapy begins, and practicing skills and tasks that are assigned by therapists.
- Establishing realistic expectations for therapy and rehabilitation, as well as for activities of daily living, social interactions, and probability of employment.
- Addressing common misconceptions held by many patients about RSD, such as: permanent loss of function; ongoing progression of RSD that will soon affect their whole body; resting an affected limb if it is painful instead of using it or exercising through the pain.
- While in therapy patients should be focusing on pain management and not cure and

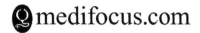

that the skills they are learning will help them be proactive and be able to better manage the pain. While the RSD may pass or abate for some patients, there are many who continue to suffer symptoms and need encouragement to stay positive and in control of their situation.

Psychological Assessment

The key psychological issues that will impact treatment and should, therefore, be evaluated include:

- Presence of coexisting psychiatric disorders that are common in RSD patients, such as major depression, panic disorder, generalized anxiety disorder, or post-traumatic stress disorder. Estimates are that up to one in four patients with RSD may suffer from one of these disorders, with depression being the most common comorbidity. These conditions impact significantly on the treatment of RSD due to the resulting lack of motivation which is a key ingredient necessary for self-management skills.
- Identification of the areas of stress in the patient's life.
- The response of close family members to the patient with RSD.
- How the patient responds to pain and to fear of pain, level of bracing or disuse, and overall functioning.
- How the patient copes with sensory abnormalities (allodynia and hyperesthesia)

As these issues are evaluated during the psychological assessment, the health care professional should communicate the relevant issues to the various members of the rehabilitation team so that team members can integrate their therapy to address these issues.

Pain Management Skills

Many patients harbor cognitive misconceptions regarding pain and progression in RSD. Common false assumptions include:

- RSD is always progressive, spreads throughout the body, and is untreatable
- If there is pain, then the affected limb has been damaged and the limb should not be used
- Treatments that cause pain and may progress slowly should not be pursued; rather interventional therapies should provide a "quick fix"

One of the most widely used techniques for teaching patients how to stay "in control" of their RSD and develop skills to manage their pain is *Cognitive Behavioral Therapy* (CBT). Cognitive Behavioral Therapy focuses on changing patients' cognitive patterns (thoughts) as a means of changing their behavior or emotional states. The premise in CBT is that a person's own thoughts cause feelings and behaviors, rather than external factors such as people or events. With CBT, patients are taught to change the way they think in order to feel better even if the situation around them does not change. For example, in the face of fear of pain or using a limb which they have been not using (bracing or guarding from pain), patients would be taught to say to himself or herself "I can handle this" or "I won't know if I can handle this until I try". They can test the cognitive skills they have learned when going to physical, occupational, or recreational therapy. These new cognitive skills can also be practiced at home repeatedly, giving patients the feeling of success by seeing how they can begin to make small steps of improvement that they could not do before.

Cognitive behavior therapy is a labor-intensive therapy with a lot of talking, thinking, examining, and integrating cognitive changes, but it is highly effective in controlling chronic pain over time and managing emotional and psychological responses to other symptoms of RSD. Cognitive Behavioral Therapy is also a time-limited therapy that continues for 12-16 sessions. At therapy termination, the patient should have learned to think differently and be able to act and respond to pain with that new thinking mode. Patients need to understand that the skills they have learned are important even if they do not experience full recovery, since the primary goal of therapy is pain management and resolution of pain is an added benefit.

Negative thoughts, discouragement, depression and anxiety all are counterproductive to progress in therapy for RSD and can actually exacerbate the condition. Patients' thoughts and behavior patterns can affect symptoms and level of disability and can be an impediment to recovery and coping with pain. Cognitive Behavioral Therapy shifts their thinking away from pain, helps them figure out how to acknowledge and cope with their pain, and then to focus on positive aspects of life. It helps reduce stress related to pain and prepares the mind and body to respond when episodes of pain occur. It also teaches patients how to become more active and take charge over their pain. Feeling calmer when confronted with pain gives patients more energy and the resources to deal with the pain.

Other therapies which may be initiated to enhance the effectiveness of CBT include:

- Biofeedback
- Relaxation therapy

Biofeedback

Biofeedback enables patients with RSD to increase control of their symptoms, which then impacts on the negative emotions and stress that affect RSD. *Biofeedback* is a technique that trains individuals to improve their health through auditory or visual feedback provided by their own bodies.

Biofeedback is typically performed on patients with RSD to promote relaxation for

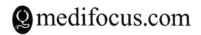

symptoms such as:

- "Protective" guarding or bracing of an extremity or of a muscle group - as the patient is taught how to use the feedback to relax a limb, blood flow to the limb increases and numerous benefits ensue, including reduced pain. Although the mechanism is not clearly understood, biofeedback appears to help many patients gain some measure of control over their pain.
- RSD-related anxiety disorders - the patient learns how to replace brain waves associated with stress with those of relaxation.
- Cooler temperature of the affected limb - through biofeedback training, the patient can be taught to raise the temperature of the limb, which also reflects increased blood flow and all of its benefits.

Biofeedback must be practiced daily in order to be effective and learning to do it effectively requires patience and persistence. Patience is also required until it actually takes effect and one experiences the reduction of pain.

Relaxation Therapy

Relaxation therapy includes techniques that induce a calming of the mind and body through mental or physical relaxation. The goals of relaxation therapy are to control pain, improve function, and enhance the patient's feelings of well-being. The process of relaxation therapy also helps to facilitate a change in attitude enabling the patient to work harder in physical therapy and raise the levels of pain tolerance.

Relaxation therapy techniques that may help RSD patients include:

- Deep breathing exercises
- Meditation
- Visual imagery
- Hypnosis
- Yoga
- Tai chi

Additional Treatments for Reflex Sympathetic Dystrophy

Additional treatments for reflex sympathetic dystrophy (RSD) that may be used alone or combined with the treatments mentioned above include:

Topical Medications

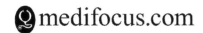

There are very few clinical trials investigating topical medications in RSD; however, there is anecdotal evidence that topical lidocaine may be effective for pain relief for some people with RSD. A variety of pain medications (e.g., lidocaine, fentanyl, and clonidine) are available as adhesive patches that release the drug over an extended period of time for alleviation of pain. Due to potential side-effects of some of these drugs, the pain patches may be appropriate only for a subset of RSD patients.

Transcutaneous Electrical Nerve Stimulation (TENS)

Transcutaneous electrical nerve stimulation, also known as TENS, is a noninvasive treatment that sends an electrical current to nerves over a specific area to relieve pain, reduce stiffness, and improve mobility. A typical TENS unit consists of an electrical signal generator, a battery, and a set of electrodes. The electrode patches are placed on the skin over the area to be treated and a mild current is generated from the stimulator controlled by the patient. Portable TENS units are available for self-treatment with a small battery-operated stimulator that can be worn around the waist. The patient can turn the stimulator on or off as needed for pain control. It is important for a health care provider, such as a physical therapist, to carefully instruct the patient on the proper use and care of the TENS unit, especially the correct placement of the electrodes. Complications of TENS units are rare, with skin irritation at the site of electrode placement being the most common side-effect.

Contraindications to the use of a TENS unit include:

- Patients with an implanted pacemaker
- Women who are pregnant (risk of premature labor)
- Patients with medical conditions that involve sensory impairment such as neuropathy or numbness, since heated electrodes could cause burns of which patients may not be aware.

Acupuncture

Acupuncture may provide temporary pain relief in some RSD patients. Adverse effects may include:

- Bleeding
- Skin irritation
- Inflammation
- Poor wound healing
- Nerve irritation and/or injury
- Intensification of pain

Trigger Point Injections

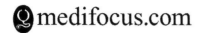

Trigger points are tender muscles that cause pain locally or in another area of the body when they are palpated or touched. A trigger point injection involves injection of a local anesthetic such as lidocaine or a corticosteroid medication into the trigger point to control and reduce pain.

Amputation

There is very little information in the medical literature about amputation as a treatment modality for RSD. Amputation is rarely performed as a treatment for RSD but may be considered under extreme circumstances, including:

- Unremitting or uncontrolled pain who refractory to medical and surgical therapy (sympathectomy)
- Recurrent infection of the RSD-affected limb
- Patients with severe RSD who have significant functional impairment

A study published in 1995 in the *British Journal of Bone and Joint Surgery* (vol. 77(2):270-3) reported on the outcomes of amputation in 28 patients with RSD. Of the five patients with untenable pain, amputation only relieved the pain in two of these patients. In contrast, amputation was found to be a relatively effective treatment for patients with recurrent infections or as a means of improving residual limb function. The authors of the study noted that recurrence of RSD in the stump following amputation occurred in most of these patients.

Repetitive Transcranial Magnetic Stimulation

Repetitive transcranial magnetic stimulation (rTMS) of the motor cortex is being studied as a way of reducing the intensity of pain association with RSD for some patients. The results of a small randomized clinical trial published in 2004 in *Neuroscience Letters* (vol. 356(2):87-90) involving ten patients with RSD reported promising results with respect to reduced pain intensity in seven of ten patients who were treated with this technique.

Hyperbaric Oxygen Therapy

Hyperbaric oxygen (HBO) therapy involves placing a patient into a special chamber called a *hyperbaric chamber* into which oxygen, under higher pressure than in the environment, is pumped. Hyperbaric oxygen therapy is currently used to treat a variety of different conditions including decompression sickness, carbon monoxide poisoning, and certain types of soft-tissue infections. The results of a small clinical trial published in 2004 in *Journal of International Medical Research* (vol. 32(3):258-62) involving 37 patients reported that HBO therapy was an effective and well-tolerated treatment for decreasing pain and swelling and increasing the range of motion for patients with RSD, but those results have not been replicated.

Progression of Treatment for Reflex Sympathetic Dystrophy

Following a diagnosis of reflex sympathetic dystrophy (RSD), there are varying opinions among clinicians regarding the progression of treatment. The overall consensus among most Guidelines published for the treatment of RSD is that treatment should begin with education of the patient about RSD, restoration of function of the affected limb through physical and occupational therapy, and strong encouragement to use the limb. If adjunct treatment is necessary to enable the patient to tolerate or ease the pain of RSD in order to proceed with therapy, then medication, nerve block or spinal cord stimulation should be considered. Hydrotherapy is especially helpful for rehabilitation of patients with RSD of the lower extremities. Increasingly interventional therapies should be considered only for patients who are refractory to all treatment and whose quality of life and function is severely affected by RSD, in conjunction with psychological counseling and Cognitive Behavioral Therapy. The employment of Cognitive Behavioral Therapy simultaneously with functional restoration appears to be particularly beneficial for children. While it is generally recognized that RSD must be treated aggressively, caution should be taken to ensure that the therapy will not be harmful for the patient.

Treatment of Myofascial Pain in Reflex Sympathetic Dystrophy

Myofascial pain and trigger points should be treated aggressively. Management of this painful aspect of RSD is usually addressed and incorporated into the various therapies used to treat reflex sympathetic dystrophy (RSD). The Reflex Sympathetic Dystrophy Syndrome Association (RSDSA) notes that treatments that are effective for myofascial pain include:

- Stretching exercises and correcting postural changes (these are considered to be crucial components of any treatment program for myofascial pain)
- Injection therapy with agents that include local anesthetics, steroids and/or saline, or botulinum toxin A (Botox)
- Application of heat and ice
- Acupuncture
- Biofeedback

Treatment of Reflex Sympathetic Dystrophy in Children and Adolescents

Treatment options for children with reflex sympathetic dystrophy (RSD) have not

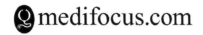

undergone rigorous clinical trials. Children appear to respond to intensive physical therapy but there is also benefit to be derived from multidisciplinary treatment. Some children respond to *transcutaneous electric nerve stimulation* (TENS) and it is considered worthwhile as a treatment option due to its safety and its acceptance by children. As with adults, treatment decisions for children with RSD should have the objective of providing the opportunity for the child to participate in rehabilitation and tolerate aggressive physical therapy. There are no randomized trials studying efficacy of medication in children and many clinicians try to avoid their use due to adverse effects. Some clinicians use sympathetic nerve blocks to facilitate rehabilitation. It is important for the timing of the treatment to be coordinated with a patient's physical therapist in order to take advantage of the available window of opportunity for aggressive treatment. Spinal cord stimulation may be effective for children and is preferable to sympathectomy since it is reversible and nondestructive. Sympathectomy may be reserved for children who are refractory to other treatment and who may lose function because of coexisting symptoms.

It is generally thought that children do not necessarily have an easier course of RSD than adults and they may be more willing to tolerate more intensive physical therapy resulting in relief or recovery from symptoms. The rate of recurrence of RSD among children and adolescents is thought to be higher than for adults; however, they respond well with the initiation of treatment.

For more in-depth information about RSD in children and adolescents, please click on the following link: http://www.ncbi.nlm.nih.gov/pubmed/16772799

Treatment of Reflex Sympathetic Dystrophy in Stroke Patients

The principle of mobilizing the limb and increasing range of motion through physical therapy is the same for RSD in stroke patients as for RSD in non-stroke patients. However, since there is a high correlation in post-stroke patients between shoulder dysfunction and RSD, physical therapy also should focus on:

- Increasing range of motion of the shoulder joint
- Strengthening the shoulder muscles
- Reducing spasticity of the shoulder muscles

Several studies have shown that mirror therapy is particularly effective for treatment of upper limb RSD in post-stroke patients.

A study published in 2000 noted that when inpatient rehabilitation was initiated at an early stage after stroke onset, the incidence of RSD in the study subjects was approximately

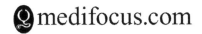

1-2%. The authors conclude the incidence of RSD in patients who do not undergo early inpatient rehabilitation is higher and may be reflected in the 12% incidence that is generally noted in the literature for post-stroke RSD. However, RSD can develop if the goals set for physical therapy are not carried out on a consistent basis after the patient is discharged from rehabilitation services.

For more information about the prevention of RSD through early rehabilitation following stroke, please click on the following link: http://www.ncbi.nlm.nih.gov/pubmed/11228950

Prognosis for Reflex Sympathetic Dystrophy

The prognosis for reflex sympathetic dystrophy (RSD) is unpredictable. Prognosis is typically better with earlier diagnosis and treatment. While some people experience spontaneous remission within the first 2-3 months, others may require intensive therapy before they experience relief, while others suffer for many years with pain and residual symptoms. Multidisciplinary rehabilitation appears to be an effective protocol for many people, and includes functional rehabilitation with intensive physical therapy; drug therapy and interventional treatment initiated on an "as-needed" basis to facilitate functional rehabilitation; psychological/behavioral therapy to provide patients with skills to manage their pain during and after therapy while reducing the impact on their quality of life. Patients who are refractory to treatment may be candidates for interventional therapies such as nerve block or sympathectomy.

The rate of recurrence of RSD is unknown, although it is thought to occur in up to 10% of patients. Recurrence can affect the same limb or a contralateral limb. A recent study that was published in 2009 in *Injury* (vol.40(8):901-4) investigated the quality of life in adults who had been treated for childhood-onset RSD. The median follow-up period was 12 years. Results indicated that the prognosis for childhood-onset RSD is not as favorable as reported in earlier literature and is comparable to the prognosis of patients with adult-onset RSD, namely a decreased quality of life and a large percentage of relapse (approximately 33%) at long-term follow-up.

Patients who experience a significant impact on their lifestyle and quality of life not only have to cope with severe pain and other related symptoms, but they also may have to cope with physical limitations, restricted social activity, unemployment, trouble sleeping, guilt, change of role in the family, and other issues. It is understandable that depression and anxiety are common comorbidities (coexisting medical conditions) for people coping with RSD. Management of their symptoms may require several professionals, such as pain specialist, psychiatrist, psychologist, physical therapist, or occupational therapist.

Epidemiological Survey of Reflex Sympathetic

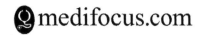

Dystrophy

Unfortunately, RSD remains a poorly understood disorder and critical information about many aspects of the disorder including its epidemiology, pathophysiology, and optimal treatment is still lacking. In order to gain a better understanding of the disorder, researchers from Columbia University (New York, NY), Johns Hopkins University (Baltimore, MD) and the Reflex Sympathetic Dystrophy Syndrome Association of America (RSDSA) conducted a Web-based cross-sectional survey and gathered data pertaining to the epidemiology, symptomology, treatment, and psychological factors related to RSD. The researchers devised a survey consisting of 75 questions and posted the survey on the RSDSA website for a five-month period from October 2004 to February 2005. The results of this study were published in 2008 in *Regional Anesthesia and Pain Medicine* (Volume 34, Issue 2; pp. 110-115).

A total of 1,359 visitors to the RSDSA website completed the survey. Of these, 888 subjects met the inclusion criteria for RSD and served as the study population for the data analysis. A summary of the major findings of the survey is presented below:

Survey Results for Onset and Presentation of RSD
- Trauma/injury was reported as the underlying "trigger" of RSD by all 888 subjects. The most common types of precipitating traumatic events or injuries reported were:

  - surgery
  - fractures
  - sprains
  - crush injuries

- The most commonly reported symptoms associated with the onset of RSD included:

  - temperature changes
  - swelling
  - color changes
  - skin changes
  - motor weakness
  - sweat changes
  - nail changes

- The average intensity of the pain associated with RSD, on a rating scale of 0 to 10, was 8.2. The pain was frequently described by subjects as:

  - burning

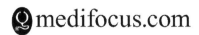

- sharp
- aching or throbbing
- stabbing

- The most commonly reported sites of pain were the lower (56%) and upper (38%) extremities. Less frequently reported sites of pain included the face, head, stomach, or back.

- Subjects had visited an average of five doctors before the diagnosis of RSD was made and an average of four doctors before treatment and follow-up was established.

Survey Results for Course and Progression of RSD

- Most subjects reported experiencing additional symptoms at the site of initial RSD involvement after the disease onset. Most commonly, these symptoms included:

  - sudomotor changes
  - trophic changes
  - motor changes
  - hypoesthesia or loss of sensation

- 80% of subjects reported that the symptoms of RSD had spread from the site of initial involvement to a new site.

- 21% of subjects reported a remission of their symptoms at some point during the course of their disease.
- 16% of subjects reported being pain-free at the time they completed the survey.
- The average intensity of daily pain (on a rating scale of 0 to 10) improved from 8.2 at the time of initial onset of RSD to 6.9 at the time of the survey.
- Subjects reported experiencing a worsening of their pain under the following conditions:

  - physical stress
  - cold weather
  - movement of the RSD-affected limb
  - work
  - emotional stress

- Predominant symptoms for most subjects at the time of the survey included:

  - temperature differences
  - hypersensitivity
  - swelling

- 18% of subjects reported being disabled at the time of the survey.

- Subjects reported that the pain associated with RSD affected their:

  - sleep
  - activities of daily living
  - mobility
  - self-care

- Approximately 75% of subjects reported feelings of anxiety and depression and 49% reported having suicidal ideations at some point during the course of their RSD. Fifteen percent of subjects with suicidal ideations had actually attempted to commit suicide.

Survey Results for Treatments for RSD

- Typically, most subjects had attempted both pharmacological and non-pharmacological therapies in an effort to control their RSD symptoms.
- Improvement of RSD symptoms was reported by subjects with the following medications:

  - intravenous lidocaine
  - opioids
  - homeopathic medications
  - DMSO cream
  - topical lidocaine
  - NSAIDs

- At the time of the survey, the most commonly reported non-pharmacological treatments used by subjects included:

  - counseling
  - physical therapy
  - spinal cord stimulation
  - nerve blocks
  - occupational therapy
  - intrathecal drug delivery

- In general, subjects reported that the level of benefit of non-pharmacological therapies for the control of their RSD symptoms ranged from "moderate" to "good".

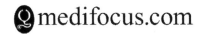

For more information about this study, please click on the following link:
http://www.ncbi.nlm.nih.gov/pubmed/19282709

Quality of Life Issues in Reflex Sympathetic Dystrophy

Reflex sympathetic dystrophy (RSD) can be a lifelong condition that can have a significant impact not only on the patient but on family and friends as well. The condition may affect many aspects of the patient's life in varying degrees including:

- Activities of daily living
- Employment
- Social life
- Personal life

Some of the adjustments of daily life that the patient may have to make include:

- Frequent leave of absence from work or possibly early retirement due to inability or difficulty performing work-related tasks
- Giving up or modifying leisure activities such as hiking, kayaking, traveling
- Modification of exercise regimens
- Foregoing routine activities such as driving or shopping
- Participating in family activities and outings

Quality of life issues among patients with chronic RSD are related to:

- Chores around the house
- Jobs (employment)
- Holidays
- Hobbies
- Social life
- Sex life

Patients with chronic RSD of the upper extremity report that chronic pain, difficulty sleeping, and lack of energy were the most distressing aspects of the condition that impacted on their quality of life. Mobility was not a significant issue for these patients. The greatest disruptions in daily life appear to be related to:

- Hobbies
- Household chores
- Self care
- Employment

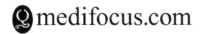

The overall quality of life scores for patients with chronic RSD are lower than for patients with diabetics, people with migraine headache, and people with chronic lung disease, all of whom traditionally report significant disruption in their quality of life.

Reflex sympathetic dystrophy may create a financial strain on patients and their families due to reduced income, unemployment, and additional medical expenses required for various treatments. It may be prudent for patients and their families to meet with a financial planner and/or an insurance agent to devise a budget to account for eventual and unexpected expenses. This may reduce the general stress level for patients and their loved ones.

Friends and family may find it beneficial to map out a plan of action with the patient's participation so that a daily routine is established. This reduces stress levels and minimizes unexpected changes in plans. Responsibilities that may need to be addressed include:

- Planning meals
- Cooking
- Cleaning
- Laundry
- Shopping
- Car pools
- Pet care
- Leisure activities

Psychosocial Issues in Reflex Sympathetic Dystrophy

Because currently there is no cure for reflex sympathetic dystrophy (RSD), the disorder may persist for a prolonged period of time and can have a significant psychosocial impact on patients. The chronic, severe nature of pain experienced by many RSD patients, particularly those with established and long-standing RSD, may lead to psychological comorbidities including depression, anxiety, feelings of isolation, and a sense of hopelessness and helplessness. In some cases, patients may be at increased the risk of suicide or thoughts of suicide. It is, therefore, important for patients and their families to recognize and understand the potential psychological effects of RSD and seek a thorough psychological consultation and evaluation as part of the overall strategy for managing RSD.

A variety of different treatment options are available to help RSD patients with concurrent psychological comorbidity including drug therapy and Cognitive Behavioral Therapy. A multidisciplinary approach to treatment involving a pain management specialist,

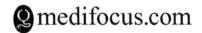
neurologist, physiatrist (specialist in physical medicine and rehabilitation), and/or a psychologist or psychiatrist may be necessary to help RSD patients learn to better cope and adjust to both the physical and psychological consequences of the disorder.

Because RSD is so poorly understood, there are physicians who are not familiar with the condition and its symptoms who perceive their patients' complaints to be psychiatric in nature ("it's all in your head"). Also, since RSD is related to many cases of worker's compensation for an injury occurring on the job, there may be a tendency for some health care providers to view patients' complaints as malingering. This is a significant source of stress for many patients and may lead to delays in diagnosis and treatment. This situation adds to the psychosocial issues patients already deal with due to chronic pain and interruption in their quality of life.

Some patients become depressed if their condition prevents them from doing things that are important to their independence and well being. Formerly independent people may have to rely on others for daily tasks, (e.g., dressing, cooking, and errands) which is inconvenient and may also feel is also demeaning, robbing them of self-respect. It is important for patients and health care providers to address these feelings and to respond to them effectively. It is hard for many patients to accept their changing condition and they actually go through a grieving process in the course of coming to terms with their new reality.

The medical literature describes four stages through which people move in relating to chronic pain:

- Hoping that there is some cure that will make the pain go away
- Wondering if the treatment they are receiving is appropriate
- Feeling anger, resentment, or depression when they realize the pain is not temporary
- Evaluating changes in lifestyle as they accept that permanent pain and varying levels of disability is their new reality

Family and friends who form the support group around patients must be educated and made aware of these reactions and should be encouraged to learn about the supporting role they can play. They need to understand what patients are going through and allow patients the opportunity to express their grief and frustration without being judgmental. Family and friends also need to be supportive and encourage patients to keep their spirits up and to continue functioning to the best of their ability.

Attitude and self-perception are crucial factors for continuing to maintain a good quality of life. As patients struggle with their situation they may be beset by feelings of inadequacy and worthlessness. Some of the following activities may be beneficial:

- Keeping a journal
- Setting goals (e.g., daily, weekly, monthly)
- Exercising (with the guidance of various therapists and physicians)
- Getting involved with a spiritual or religious group
- Reading
- Volunteering
- Counseling

Despite a wide range of treatment options available to patients with RSD, some patients do not seek help since they may be discouraged by constant pain and are worn down both physically and emotionally. This may result in their dismissing efforts by others to help them. Some of their concerns include:

- Fear that nothing can help them
- Fear that they will become addicted to medications
- Fear that they will be seen as "complainers" if they complain about their pain
- Fear of side effects of treatments
- Fear that they will develop a tolerance to medications and that the recurring pain will be even worse

It is important to discuss these concerns with family members, friends, physicians, and/or support service professionals (e.g., psychologist, social worker) in order to take advantage of options that are available and may actually lead to pain relief and/or improvement in the overall quality of life.

Patients should be encouraged to join a support group or to seek psychological counseling if necessary. Patients may even reach the point of ultimately counseling others with RSD. Some patients find benefit in getting involved in volunteer work which allows them to set their own hours and to feel that they still can contribute to others instead of just focusing on their own condition.

Lifestyle Modifications in Reflex Sympathetic Dystrophy

In order to remain as independent as possible and to minimize the disruption of daily life, individuals with reflex sympathetic dystrophy (RSD) may need to consider changes and modifications that need to be made not only in their daily routine but in their surroundings as well. For example, for the person with lower extremity RSD, getting around can cause a significant challenge since normal activities (e.g., walking, climbing stairs, sitting for long periods of time with knees flexed, and getting in and out of cars) can be quite painful. Patients and their families should assess their surroundings, perhaps with the help of

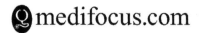

professionals (such as an occupational therapist), and prioritize the modifications that will help them maintain their independence and function.

Some of the modifications in their surroundings that patients with RSD may wish to consider include:

Clothing

- Velcro or zippers instead of shoelaces
- Slip-on shoes
- Flat shoes instead of heels for patients with lower extremity RSD
- Velcro or zipper closures for shirts or sweaters

Bathroom

- Grab bars in the bathtub, shower, and next to the toilet
- Tub or shower bench
- Long-handle comb or brush to avoid raising the arm too high
- Elevated toilet seat

Kitchen

- Large knobs on appliances requiring manipulation (e.g., stove, dishwasher, washing machine)
- Easy-grab handles for cabinets
- Lightweight dishes and pots
- Lightweight flatware with long handles
- Sliding shelves or turntables on kitchen shelves so the patient does not have to reach into cabinets to access items at the back of a shelf
- Long handled cleaning appliances, (e.g., brooms, dustpans, sponges)
- Lightweight appliances (e.g., vacuum cleaner)
- Long-handled "grabbers" for removing items on high shelves or picking up items from the floor

Bedroom

- Blanket support frame so that blankets or sheets do not rest directly on the feet of a patient with allodynia
- Nightlights in the bedroom and any other rooms where patients may walk if they awaken during the night

Automobile

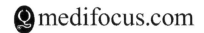
- Modified controls to facilitate driving
- Car doors that are easy to open and close
- Seat positions that are easy to manipulate
- Handicapped parking stickers

Miscellaneous

- Voice-activated lights, appliances, or computer
- Electric wheelchair to avoid upper body strain or injury
- Wheelchair-access modifications at home
- Nursing or home health care
- Physician-recommended special accommodations, such as an aisle seat in airplanes
- Use of wheelchairs in airports, train stations, or malls
- Medical support professionals and/or accountants to budget for medications, special appliances, home-nursing care, and other medical related supplies and expenses

Maintaining a Healthy Lifestyle in Reflex Sympathetic Dystrophy

It is important for the patient with reflex sympathetic dystrophy (RSD) to maintain a healthy lifestyle despite the difficulties they are experiencing, including getting enough sleep, exercising, and eating healthy foods. Patients must be particularly vigilant about the potential long-term health consequences of a changing life style caused by chronic pain. Since patients with RSD may be forced to lead a more sedentary lifestyle, they may be more at risk for developing other medical problems including:

- Weight gain
- Cardiovascular disease
- Osteoporosis
- Diabetes

Weight control is crucial for overall good health in addition to eating balanced meals (including dietary supplements or vitamins if needed). It is also beneficial to find facilities that offer modified exercise programs for physically handicapped individuals. For individuals who have a tendency to shield the affected limb from any stimulation or from being touched or manipulated, it is very important to maintain hygiene of the affected limb even though it it may be perceived as being painful.

Sleep Disturbances in Reflex Sympathetic

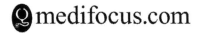

Dystrophy

Sleep disturbances due to chronic, severe pain of reflex sympathetic dystrophy (RSD) can have a significant detrimental effect on quality of life. Sleep deficit can actually prolong pain for patients with RSD in addition to affecting mood, level of fatigue, and ability to function well in activities of daily living. It has been estimated that approximately 50-70% of people with chronic pain experience sleep disturbances. If sleep is an issue for the RSD patient, it is important to communicate this concern to a health care provider. Some techniques the patient may try include taking a nap early in the day instead of late afternoon and avoiding nicotine, caffeine, and alcohol. A variety of treatment options are available for RSD patients who experience chronic sleep disturbances, including medications and psychological interventions, and these options should be discussed with patients'health care provider.

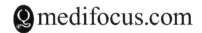medifocus.com

New Developments in Reflex Sympathetic Dystrophy

- Researchers in Australia are studying the efficacy of topical ketamine for the relief of sensory disturbances associated with RSD. Results of a small study published in November 2009 show promise; but additional studies are needed. To read about topical ketamine and RSD, please click on the following link: http://www.ncbi.nlm.nih.gov/pubmed/19703730

- A small study was published investigating the efficacy of motor cortex electrical stimulation applied to patients with RSD who were unresponsive to all medical treatment. Pre- and post-operative evaluations were carried out monthly for one year and changes in pain as well as sensory and sympathetic symptoms (temperature, perspiration, color, and swelling) were evaluated. Four of the five patients showed significant decreases in pain, sensory, and sympathetic changes, while one patient showed no improvement. Further trials are needed to confirm these findings. For more information about this study, please click on the following link: http://www.ncbi.nlm.nih.gov/pubmed/19793621

- A study published by researchers in the Netherlands in February 2010 reported that a higher level of brush-evoked allodynia (abnormal sensations caused by the stroke of a brush on the skin) in patients with RSD may be a significant negative prognostic indicator of the successful outcome of spinal cord stimulation (SCS) one year after treatment. Since SCS is an invasive and relatively expensive treatment for RSD, prognostic factors may be important factors to consider before proceeding with the treatment. Further studies are planned. To read more about this, please click on the following link: http://www.ncbi.nlm.nih.gov/pubmed/19942463

- Investigation continues regarding the possibility of an autoimmune mechanism in the development of RSD which could ultimately influence treatment for this condition. Tumor necrosis factor (TNF)-alpha, which has been detected in many immunologically based diseases, has also been detected in the affected hands of three patients diagnosed with early-stage RSD. For more information, please click on the following link: http://www.ncbi.nlm.nih.gov/pubmed/19910617

- There is evidence from several studies that a daily dose of 500 mg of vitamin C may prevent development of RSD if initiated as soon as the diagnosis of a wrist fracture is determined. In addition, vitamin C has been shown to be effective in preventing RSD when taken prior to surgery of the foot and ankle. For more information about vitamin C and RSD, please click on the following link:

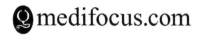

http://www.ncbi.nlm.nih.gov/pubmed/19840748

- A study published in *Disability and Rehabilitation* in 2009 evaluated the effects of intramuscular injections of calcitonin in preventing RSD in post-stroke patients with severe hemiplegia. One group of patients received the injections weekly together with rehabilitation therapy while the other group (control group) received rehabilitation only. Results indicated that the onset of RSD was approximately 8% in the control group. RSD was completely prevented when the injections were initiated four weeks or less following a stroke, but that the effect was much weaker if injections were started more than six weeks after stroke. To read more about this study, please click on the following link:
http://www.ncbi.nlm.nih.gov/pubmed/19479511

- A pilot study was published exploring the feasibility of magnesium infusions as a treatment for RSD. Eight patients participated in the study and received infusions for five days. Follow-up at 12 weeks showed that there was a significant improvement in pain, level of impairment, and quality of life. The treatment was well tolerated. There was no improvement in allodynia or functional limitations. Larger studies are recommended to confirm these findings. To read more about this study, please click on the following link: http://www.ncbi.nlm.nih.gov/pubmed/19496957

- Investigators at Drexel University College of Medicine in Philadelphia, PA assessed the relative frequency of migraine headaches and headache characteristics of 124 patients with RSD. The conclusion they reached was that migraine headaches may be a risk factor for RSD and that the presence of migraine headache may be associated with a more severe form of RSD. To read about more specific findings of the relationship between migraine headache and RSD, please click on the following link: http://www.ncbi.nlm.nih.gov/pubmed/19614690

- A pilot study was published in the *Clinical Journal of Pain* regarding the efficacy of a drug called *Memantine* in patients with RSD. Results from this small study indicate a reduction in the level of pain, an improvement of motor symptoms, and improvement of autonomic changes. To read more about this study, please click on the following link: http://www.ncbi.nlm.nih.gov/pubmed/17314583

- If you are interested in information about clinical trials for RSD, please visit http://www.clinicaltrials.gov.

Questions to Ask Your Health Care Provider about Reflex Sympathetic Dystrophy

- How can you be certain that I have reflex sympathetic dystrophy (RSD) and not another chronic pain condition?
- What treatments do you recommend and why?
- What are my treatment options?
- In your experience, is there a "best" treatment?
- What is my prognosis (short and long term)?
- Are there any activities I can be doing on my own to either improve my condition or prevent it from getting worse?
- At what point do you recommend interventional therapies?
- Which other health care professionals should be involved in my treatment?
- Is the proposed treatment covered by my health insurance policy?
- How much experience have you had treating patients with RSD?
- Are there any doctors in the area that specialize in managing RSD patients?
- Are there any RSD support groups in this area?

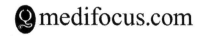

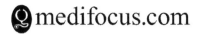

NOTES

Use this page for taking notes as you review your Guidebook

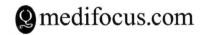

3 - Guide to the Medical Literature

Introduction

This section of your *MediFocus Guidebook* is a comprehensive bibliography of important recent medical literature published about the condition from authoritative, trustworthy medical journals. This is the same information that is used by physicians and researchers to keep up with the latest advances in clinical medicine and biomedical research. A broad spectrum of articles is included in each *MediFocus Guidebook* to provide information about standard treatments, treatment options, new developments, and advances in research.

To facilitate your review and analysis of this information, the articles in this *MediFocus Guidebook* are grouped in the following categories:

- Review Articles - 62 Articles
- General Interest Articles - 79 Articles
- Drug Therapy Articles - 13 Articles
- Clinical Trials Articles - 30 Articles
- Nerve Block Articles - 5 Articles
- Electrical Stimulation Articles - 10 Articles

The following information is provided for each of the articles referenced in this section of your *MediFocus Guidebook:*

- Title of the article
- Name of the authors
- Institution where the study was done
- Journal reference (Volume, page numbers, year of publication)
- Link to Abstract (brief summary of the actual article)

Linking to Abstracts: Most of the medical journal articles referenced in this section of your *MediFocus Guidebook* include an abstract (brief summary of the actual article) that can be accessed online via the National Library of Medicine's PubMed® database. You can easily access the individual article abstracts online by entering the individual URL address for a particular article into your web browser, or by going to the following special URL:

http://www.medifocus.com/links/NR015/0314

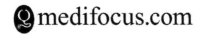

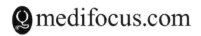

Recent Literature: What Your Doctor Reads

Database: PubMed <January 2009 to March 2014>

Review Articles

1.

Imaging and clinical evidence of sensorimotor problems in CRPS: utilizing novel treatment approaches.

Authors:	Bailey J; Nelson S; Lewis J; McCabe CS
Institution:	Bath Centre for Pain Services, The Royal National Hospital for Rheumatic Diseases, Upper Borough Walls, Bath BA1 1RL, UK.
Journal:	J Neuroimmune Pharmacol. 2013 Jun;8(3):564-75. doi: 10.1007/s11481-012-9405-9. Epub 2012 Oct 11.
Abstract Link:	http://www.medifocus.com/abstracts.php?gid=NR015&ID=23054370

2.

Treatment of complex regional pain syndrome in adults: a systematic review of randomized controlled trials published from June 2000 to February 2012.

Authors:	Cossins L; Okell RW; Cameron H; Simpson B; Poole HM; Goebel A
Institution:	Pain Research Institute, Clinical Sciences Centre, University Hospital Aintree, Liverpool, UK.
Journal:	Eur J Pain. 2013 Feb;17(2):158-73. doi: 10.1002/j.1532-2149.2012.00217.x. Epub 2012 Oct 5.
Abstract Link:	http://www.medifocus.com/abstracts.php?gid=NR015&ID=23042687

Go to http://www.medifocus.com/links/NR015/0314 for direct online access to the above Abstract Links.

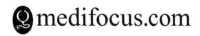medifocus.com

3.

Complex regional pain syndrome: a review.

Author:	Field J
Institution:	Cheltenham General Hospital, Cheltenham, UK. jeremy.field@glos.nhs.uk
Journal:	J Hand Surg Eur Vol. 2013 Jul;38(6):616-26. doi: 10.1177/1753193412471021. Epub 2013 Jan 22.
Abstract Link:	http://www.medifocus.com/abstracts.php?gid=NR015&ID=23340755

4.

Diagnosis of partial complex regional pain syndrome type 1 of the hand: retrospective study of 16 cases and literature review.

Authors:	Konzelmann M; Deriaz O; Luthi F
Institution:	Department for musculoskeletal rehabilitation, Clinique romande de readaptation suvacare, 90 avenue du grand champsec, Sion 1951, Switzerland. Michel.konzelmann@crr-suva.ch
Journal:	BMC Neurol. 2013 Mar 18;13:28. doi: 10.1186/1471-2377-13-28.
Abstract Link:	http://www.medifocus.com/abstracts.php?gid=NR015&ID=23506090

5.

A review of psychosocial factors in complex regional pain syndrome.

Authors:	Lohnberg JA; Altmaier EM
Institution:	Psychology Service, VA Palo Alto Health Care System, (116B), 3801 Miranda Ave., Palo Alto, CA, USA, jessica-lohnberg@uiowa.edu
Journal:	J Clin Psychol Med Settings. 2013 Jun;20(2):247-54. doi: 10.1007/s10880-012-9322-3.
Abstract Link:	http://www.medifocus.com/abstracts.php?gid=NR015&ID=22961122

Go to http://www.medifocus.com/links/NR015/0314 for direct online access to the above Abstract Links.

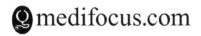

6.

Inflammation in complex regional pain syndrome: a systematic review and meta-analysis.

Authors:	Parkitny L; McAuley JH; Di Pietro F; Stanton TR; O'Connell NE; Marinus J; van Hilten JJ; Moseley GL
Institution:	Neuroscience Research Australia, University of New South Wales, Sydney, Australia.
Journal:	Neurology. 2013 Jan 1;80(1):106-17. doi: 10.1212/WNL.0b013e31827b1aa1.
Abstract Link:	http://www.medifocus.com/abstracts.php?gid=NR015&ID=23267031

7.

Efficacy and safety of high-dose vitamin C on complex regional pain syndrome in extremity trauma and surgery--systematic review and meta-analysis.

Authors:	Shibuya N; Humphers JM; Agarwal MR; Jupiter DC
Institution:	Texas A&M Health and Science Center, College of Medicine, Temple, TX, USA. shibuya@medicine.tamhsc.edu
Journal:	J Foot Ankle Surg. 2013 Jan-Feb;52(1):62-6. doi: 10.1053/j.jfas.2012.08.003. Epub 2012 Sep 15.
Abstract Link:	http://www.medifocus.com/abstracts.php?gid=NR015&ID=22985495

8.

Local anaesthetic sympathetic blockade for complex regional pain syndrome.

Authors:	Stanton TR; Wand BM; Carr DB; Birklein F; Wasner GL; O'Connell NE
Institution:	Neuroscience Research Australia, Randwick, Australia.
Journal:	Cochrane Database Syst Rev. 2013 Aug 19;8:CD004598. doi: 10.1002/14651858.CD004598.pub3.
Abstract Link:	http://www.medifocus.com/abstracts.php?gid=NR015&ID=23959684

Go to http://www.medifocus.com/links/NR015/0314 for direct online access to the above Abstract Links.

9.

Prognostic factors in complex regional pain syndrome 1: a systematic review.

Authors: Wertli M; Bachmann LM; Weiner SS; Brunner F

Institution: Horten Center for Patient Oriented Research and Knowledge Transfer, Department of Internal Medicine, University of Zurich, Pestalozzistrasse 24, CH-8032 Zurich, Switzerland.

Journal: J Rehabil Med. 2013 Mar 6;45(3):225-31. doi: 10.2340/16501977-1103.

Abstract Link: http://www.medifocus.com/abstracts.php?gid=NR015&ID=23389624

10.

Efficacy and safety of ketamine in patients with complex regional pain syndrome: a systematic review.

Authors: Azari P; Lindsay DR; Briones D; Clarke C; Buchheit T; Pyati S

Institution: Department of Anesthesiology, Division of Pain Management, Duke University School of Medicine, Durham, NC 27710, USA.

Journal: CNS Drugs. 2012 Mar 1;26(3):215-28. doi: 10.2165/11595200-000000000-00000.

Abstract Link: http://www.medifocus.com/abstracts.php?gid=NR015&ID=22136149

11.

Is physiotherapy effective for children with complex regional pain syndrome type 1?

Authors: Bialocerkowski AE; Daly A

Institution: School of Biomedical and Health Sciences, University of Western Sydney, Sydney, Australia. a.bialocerkowski@uws.edu.au

Journal: Clin J Pain. 2012 Jan;28(1):81-91.

Abstract Link: http://www.medifocus.com/abstracts.php?gid=NR015&ID=21677566

Go to http://www.medifocus.com/links/NR015/0314 for direct online access to the above Abstract Links.

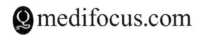

12.

Neurological diseases and pain.

Author:	Borsook D
Institution:	MD Center for Pain and the Brain C/O Brain Imaging Center, McLean Hospital Belmont, MA 02478, USA. dborsook@partners.org
Journal:	Brain. 2012 Feb;135(Pt 2):320-44. Epub 2011 Nov 8.
Abstract Link:	http://www.medifocus.com/abstracts.php?gid=NR015&ID=22067541

13.

Meta-analysis of imaging techniques for the diagnosis of complex regional pain syndrome type I.

Authors:	Cappello ZJ; Kasdan ML; Louis DS
Institution:	School of Medicine and Division of Plastic Surgery, University of Louisville, Louisville, KY, USA. zjcapp01@louisville.edu
Journal:	J Hand Surg Am. 2012 Feb;37(2):288-96. Epub 2011 Dec 15.
Abstract Link:	http://www.medifocus.com/abstracts.php?gid=NR015&ID=22177715

14.

Spinal cord stimulation: a review.

Authors:	Compton AK; Shah B; Hayek SM
Institution:	SMC Pain Center, Schneck Medical Center, 411 West Tipton Street, Seymour, IN 47274, USA.
Journal:	Curr Pain Headache Rep. 2012 Feb;16(1):35-42.
Abstract Link:	http://www.medifocus.com/abstracts.php?gid=NR015&ID=22086473

Go to http://www.medifocus.com/links/NR015/0314 for direct online access to the above Abstract Links.

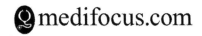 medifocus.com

15.

Effect of immunomodulating medications in complex regional pain syndrome: a systematic review.

Authors: Dirckx M; Stronks DL; Groeneweg G; Huygen FJ
Institution: Erasmus MC, Rotterdam, The Netherlands. m.dirckx@erasmusmc.nl
Journal: Clin J Pain. 2012 May;28(4):355-63.
Abstract Link: http://www.medifocus.com/abstracts.php?gid=NR015&ID=22001668

16.

Managing chronic pain with spinal cord stimulation.

Authors: Epstein LJ; Palmieri M
Institution: Department of Anesthesiology, Mount Sinai School of Medicine, New York, NY, USA. lawrence.epstein@mountsinai.org
Journal: Mt Sinai J Med. 2012 Jan-Feb;79(1):123-32. doi: 10.1002/msj.21289.
Abstract Link: http://www.medifocus.com/abstracts.php?gid=NR015&ID=22238045

17.

A review on spinal cord stimulation.

Authors: Falowski S; Sharan A
Institution: St. Lukes Neurosurgical Associates, St. Lukes University Hospital, Bethlehem, PA, USA.
Journal: J Neurosurg Sci. 2012 Dec;56(4):287-98.
Abstract Link: http://www.medifocus.com/abstracts.php?gid=NR015&ID=23111289

18.

Complex regional pain syndrome in children: asking the right questions.

Author: Goldschneider KR
Institution: Cincinnati Children's Hospital Medical Center, Cincinnati, OH, USA. kenneth.goldschneider@cchmc.org
Journal: Pain Res Manag. 2012 Nov-Dec;17(6):386-90.
Abstract Link: http://www.medifocus.com/abstracts.php?gid=NR015&ID=23248811

Go to http://www.medifocus.com/links/NR015/0314 for direct online access to the above Abstract Links.

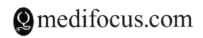
19.

Immunotherapy in miscellaneous medical disorders Graves ophthalmopathy, asthma, and regional painful syndrome.

Authors:	Gonzales M; Fratianni C; Mamillapali C; Khardori R
Institution:	Division of Endocrinology and Metabolism, Department of Internal Medicine, Strelitz Center for Diabetes and Endocrine Disorders, Eastern Virginia Medical School, 855 West Brambleton Avenue, Norfolk, VA 23510, USA.
Journal:	Med Clin North Am. 2012 May;96(3):635-54, xi.
Abstract Link:	http://www.medifocus.com/abstracts.php?gid=NR015&ID=22703859

20.

Management of soft-tissue injuries in distal radius fractures.

Authors:	Leversedge FJ; Srinivasan RC
Institution:	Department of Orthopaedic Surgery, Duke University, DUMC Box 2836, Durham, NC 27710, USA. fraser.leversedge@duke.edu
Journal:	Hand Clin. 2012 May;28(2):225-33. Epub 2012 Apr 6.
Abstract Link:	http://www.medifocus.com/abstracts.php?gid=NR015&ID=22554666

21.

Complications associated with arthroscopic rotator cuff repair: a literature review.

Authors:	Randelli P; Spennacchio P; Ragone V; Arrigoni P; Casella A; Cabitza P
Institution:	Dipartimento Di Scienze Medico-Chirurgiche, Universita Degli Studi Di Milano, IRCCS Policlinico San Donato, Milan, Italy.
Journal:	Musculoskelet Surg. 2012 Jun;96(1):9-16. doi: 10.1007/s12306-011-0175-y. Epub 2011 Dec 29.
Abstract Link:	http://www.medifocus.com/abstracts.php?gid=NR015&ID=22205384

Go to http://www.medifocus.com/links/NR015/0314 for direct online access to the above Abstract Links.

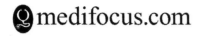

22.

Update on the pathogenesis of complex regional pain syndrome: role of oxidative stress.

Authors: Taha R; Blaise GA

Institution: Multinnova Medical Centre, Universite de Montreal, Montreal, QC, Canada.

Journal: Can J Anaesth. 2012 Sep;59(9):875-81. doi: 10.1007/s12630-012-9748-y. Epub 2012 Jul 14.

Abstract Link: http://www.medifocus.com/abstracts.php?gid=NR015&ID=22798149

23.

Chronic regional pain syndrome: what specialized rehabilitation services do patients require?

Authors: Veizi IE; Chelimsky TC; Janata JW

Institution: Departments of Psychiatry and Anesthesiology, University Hospitals Case Medical Center, Cleveland, OH 44106, USA.

Journal: Curr Pain Headache Rep. 2012 Apr;16(2):139-46. doi: 10.1007/s11916-012-0253-3.

Abstract Link: http://www.medifocus.com/abstracts.php?gid=NR015&ID=22415615

24.

Therapy-resistant complex regional pain syndrome type I: to amputate or not?

Authors: Bodde MI; Dijkstra PU; den Dunnen WF; Geertzen JH

Institution: Department of Rehabilitation Medicine, University Medical Center Groningen, P.O. Box 30.001, 9700 RB Groningen, The Netherlands. m.i.bodde@rev.umcg.nl

Journal: J Bone Joint Surg Am. 2011 Oct 5;93(19):1799-805.

Abstract Link: http://www.medifocus.com/abstracts.php?gid=NR015&ID=22005865

Go to http://www.medifocus.com/links/NR015/0314 for direct online access to the above Abstract Links.

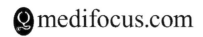
25.

Lawsuit verdicts and settlements involving reflex sympathetic dystrophy and complex regional pain syndrome.

Authors:	Crick BC; Crick JC
Institution:	North Florida Surgeons, St. Vincent's Medical Center, 1 Shircliff Way St., Jacksonville, Florida, 32204, USA.
Journal:	J Surg Orthop Adv. 2011 Fall;20(3):153-7.
Abstract Link:	http://www.medifocus.com/abstracts.php?gid=NR015&ID=22214139

26.

Complex regional pain syndrome in adults.

Author:	Goebel A
Institution:	Pain Research Group and Centre for Immune Studies in Pain, Department of Translational Medicine, University of Liverpool, UK. reasgoebel@rocketmail.com
Journal:	Rheumatology (Oxford). 2011 Oct;50(10):1739-50. Epub 2011 Jun 28.
Abstract Link:	http://www.medifocus.com/abstracts.php?gid=NR015&ID=21712368

27.

Continuous peripheral nerve blocks: a review of the published evidence.

Author:	Ilfeld BM
Institution:	Clinical Investigation, University of California San Diego, 200 West Arbor Dr., MC 8770, San Diego, CA 92103-8770, USA. bilfeld@ucsd.edu
Journal:	Anesth Analg. 2011 Oct;113(4):904-25. Epub 2011 Aug 4.
Abstract Link:	http://www.medifocus.com/abstracts.php?gid=NR015&ID=21821511

Go to http://www.medifocus.com/links/NR015/0314 for direct online access to the above Abstract Links.

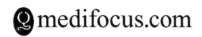

28.

Intramuscular botulinum toxin in complex regional pain syndrome: case series and literature review.

Authors:	Kharkar S; Ambady P; Venkatesh Y; Schwartzman RJ
Institution:	Hahnemann University Hospital, Philadelphia, PA and Department of Neurology, Drexel University College of Medicine, Philadelphia, PA 19107, USA.
Journal:	Pain Physician. 2011 Sep-Oct;14(5):419-24.
Abstract Link:	http://www.medifocus.com/abstracts.php?gid=NR015&ID=21927045

29.

CRPS I following artificial disc surgery: case report and review of the literature.

Authors:	Knoeller SM; Ehmer M; Kleinmann B; Wolter T
Institution:	Department of Orthopaedic and Trauma Surgery, University Hospital Freiburg, Freiburg, Germany. stefan.knoeller@uniklinik-freiburg.de
Journal:	Eur Spine J. 2011 Jul;20 Suppl 2:S278-83. Epub 2011 Jan 28.
Abstract Link:	http://www.medifocus.com/abstracts.php?gid=NR015&ID=21274730

30.

Mirror box therapy: seeing is believing.

Authors:	Lamont K; Chin M; Kogan M
Institution:	Physician Assistant Program, George Washington Center for Integrative Medicine, Washington, DC, USA.
Journal:	Explore (NY). 2011 Nov-Dec;7(6):369-72. doi: 10.1016/j.explore.2011.08.002.
Abstract Link:	http://www.medifocus.com/abstracts.php?gid=NR015&ID=22051561

Go to http://www.medifocus.com/links/NR015/0314 for direct online access to the above Abstract Links.

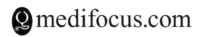

31.

Clinical features and pathophysiology of complex regional pain syndrome.

Authors: Marinus J; Moseley GL; Birklein F; Baron R; Maihofner C; Kingery WS; van Hilten JJ

Institution: Department of Neurology, Leiden University Medical Center, Leiden, Netherlands, TREND Knowledge Consortium, Leiden, Netherlands. j.marinus@lumc.nl

Journal: Lancet Neurol. 2011 Jul;10(7):637-48.

Abstract Link: http://www.medifocus.com/abstracts.php?gid=NR015&ID=21683929

32.

Complex regional pain syndrome of the upper extremity.

Authors: Patterson RW; Li Z; Smith BP; Smith TL; Koman LA

Institution: Department of Orthopaedic Surgery, Wake Forest University School of Medicine, Winston-Salem, NC 27157, USA.

Journal: J Hand Surg Am. 2011 Sep;36(9):1553-62.

Abstract Link: http://www.medifocus.com/abstracts.php?gid=NR015&ID=21872098

33.

The clinical aspects of mirror therapy in rehabilitation: a systematic review of the literature.

Authors: Rothgangel AS; Braun SM; Beurskens AJ; Seitz RJ; Wade DT

Institution: The Department of Health and Technique, Zuyd University of Applied Sciences, Heerlen, The Netherlands. a.s.rothgangel@hszuyd.nl

Journal: Int J Rehabil Res. 2011 Mar;34(1):1-13.

Abstract Link: http://www.medifocus.com/abstracts.php?gid=NR015&ID=21326041

Go to http://www.medifocus.com/links/NR015/0314 for direct online access to the above Abstract Links.

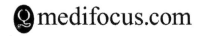

34.

The use of ketamine in complex regional pain syndrome: possible mechanisms.

Authors:	Schwartzman RJ; Alexander GM; Grothusen JR
Institution:	Department of Neurology, Drexel University College of Medicine, PA, USA. robert.schwartzman@drexelmed.edu
Journal:	Expert Rev Neurother. 2011 May;11(5):719-34.
Abstract Link:	http://www.medifocus.com/abstracts.php?gid=NR015&ID=21539489

35.

Complex regional pain syndrome.

Authors:	Shah A; Kirchner JS
Institution:	Division of Orthopaedic Surgery, University of Alabama at Birmingham, Birmingham, AL 35205-5327, USA. dr.shah.ashish@gmail.com
Journal:	Foot Ankle Clin. 2011 Jun;16(2):351-66.
Abstract Link:	http://www.medifocus.com/abstracts.php?gid=NR015&ID=21600455

36.

Complex regional pain syndrome in adults: concise guidance.

Authors:	Turner-Stokes L; Goebel A
Institution:	King's College London School of Medicine.
Journal:	Clin Med. 2011 Dec;11(6):596-600.
Abstract Link:	http://www.medifocus.com/abstracts.php?gid=NR015&ID=22268318

Go to http://www.medifocus.com/links/NR015/0314 for direct online access to the above Abstract Links.

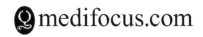

37.

An update on the pathophysiology of complex regional pain syndrome.

Author: Bruehl S
Institution: Department of Anesthesiology, Vanderbilt University School of Medicine, Nashville, Tennessee 37212, USA. stephen.bruehl@vanderbilt.edu
Journal: Anesthesiology. 2010 Sep;113(3):713-25.
Abstract Link: http://www.medifocus.com/abstracts.php?gid=NR015&ID=20693883

38.

Sensory disturbances in complex regional pain syndrome: clinical observations, autonomic interactions, and possible mechanisms.

Author: Drummond PD
Institution: School of Psychology, Murdoch University, Perth, Western Australia, Australia. P.Drummond@murdoch.edu.au
Journal: Pain Med. 2010 Aug;11(8):1257-66.
Abstract Link: http://www.medifocus.com/abstracts.php?gid=NR015&ID=20704674

39.

Psychologic factors in the development of complex regional pain syndrome: history, myth, and evidence.

Authors: Feliu MH; Edwards CL
Institution: Departments of Psychiatry double daggerHematology daggerDuke Pain and Palliative Care Clinic, Duke University Medical Center, Durham, NC 27705, USA. feliu001@mc.duke.edu
Journal: Clin J Pain. 2010 Mar-Apr;26(3):258-63.
Abstract Link: http://www.medifocus.com/abstracts.php?gid=NR015&ID=20173441

Go to http://www.medifocus.com/links/NR015/0314 for direct online access to the above Abstract Links.

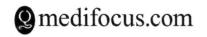

40.

Anti-inflammatory treatment of Complex Regional Pain Syndrome.

Authors: Fischer SG; Zuurmond WW; Birklein F; Loer SA; Perez RS
Institution: Department of Anesthesiology, VU University Medical Center,
                  Amsterdam, The Netherlands. s.fischer@vumc.nl
Journal: Pain. 2010 Nov;151(2):251-6. Epub 2010 Aug 7.
Abstract Link: **ABSTRACT NOT AVAILABLE**

41.

Thoracoscopic sympathectomy.

Author: Krasna MJ
Institution: Program of Health Policy, St. Joseph Cancer Institute, University of
                  Maryland, 7501 Osler Drive, Suite 104, Towson, MD 21204, USA.
                  markkrasna@catholichealth.net
Journal: Thorac Surg Clin. 2010 May;20(2):323-30.
Abstract Link: http://www.medifocus.com/abstracts.php?gid=NR015&ID=20451141

42.

Complex regional pain syndrome after hand surgery.

Authors: Li Z; Smith BP; Tuohy C; Smith TL; Andrew Koman L
Institution: Department of Orthopaedic Surgery, Wake Forest University School of
                  Medicine, Wake Forest University Health Sciences, Medical Center
                  Boulevard, Winston-Salem, NC 27157, USA.
Journal: Hand Clin. 2010 May;26(2):281-9.
Abstract Link: http://www.medifocus.com/abstracts.php?gid=NR015&ID=20494753

Go to http://www.medifocus.com/links/NR015/0314 for direct online access to the above Abstract Links.

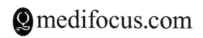

43.

Complex regional pain syndrome type I: neuropathic or not?

Authors: Naleschinski D; Baron R

Institution: Division of Neurological Pain Research and Therapy, Department of
               Neurology, University Hospital Schleswig-Holstein, Campus Kiel,
               Arnold-Heller-Str. 3, Haus 41, 24105, Kiel, Germany.
               d.naleschinski@neurologie.uni-kiel.de

Journal: Curr Pain Headache Rep. 2010 Jun;14(3):196-202.
Abstract Link: http://www.medifocus.com/abstracts.php?gid=NR015&ID=20461475

44.

What does the mechanism of spinal cord stimulation tell us about complex regional pain syndrome?

Author: Prager JP

Institution: Center for the Rehabilitation of Pain Syndromes (CRPS), UCLA
               Medical Plaza, Department of Anesthesiology, David Geffen School of
               Medicine at UCLA, Los Angeles, California 90095, USA.
               joshuaprager@gmail.com

Journal: Pain Med. 2010 Aug;11(8):1278-83.
Abstract Link: http://www.medifocus.com/abstracts.php?gid=NR015&ID=20704677

45.

Spinal cord stimulation for injured soldiers with complex regional pain syndrome.

Author: Ruamwijitphong W
Institution: DePaul Health Center, Bridgeton, MO, USA.
Journal: Nurse Pract. 2010 Aug;35(8):39-43.
Abstract Link: **ABSTRACT NOT AVAILABLE**

Go to http://www.medifocus.com/links/NR015/0314 for direct online access to the above Abstract Links.

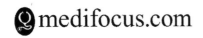
46.

Plasticity of complex regional pain syndrome (CRPS) in children.

Author: Stanton-Hicks M
Institution: Pain Management Department, Center for Neurological Restoration, Consulting Staff, Children's Hospital CCF Shaker Campus, Pediatric Pain Rehabilitation Program, Cleveland Clinic, Cleveland, Ohio 44195, USA. stantom@ccf.org
Journal: Pain Med. 2010 Aug;11(8):1216-23.
Abstract Link: http://www.medifocus.com/abstracts.php?gid=NR015&ID=20704670

47.

Cervico-thoracic or lumbar sympathectomy for neuropathic pain and complex regional pain syndrome.

Authors: Straube S; Derry S; Moore RA; McQuay HJ
Institution: Department of Occupational and Social Medicine, University of Gottingen, Waldweg 37 B, Gottingen, Germany, D-37073.
Journal: Cochrane Database Syst Rev. 2010 Jul 7;(7):CD002918.
Abstract Link: http://www.medifocus.com/abstracts.php?gid=NR015&ID=20614432

48.

Treatment of complex regional pain syndrome: a review of the evidence.

Authors: Tran de QH; Duong S; Bertini P; Finlayson RJ
Institution: Department of Anesthesia, Montreal General Hospital, McGill University, Montreal, H3G 1A4, Quebec, Canada. de_tran@hotmail.com
Journal: Can J Anaesth. 2010 Feb;57(2):149-66.
Abstract Link: http://www.medifocus.com/abstracts.php?gid=NR015&ID=20054678

Go to http://www.medifocus.com/links/NR015/0314 for direct online access to the above Abstract Links.

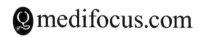

49.

Movement disorders in complex regional pain syndrome.

Author: van Hilten JJ
Institution: Department of Neurology, Leiden University Medical Center, Leiden,
                   The Netherlands. J.J.van_Hilten@lumc.nl
Journal: Pain Med. 2010 Aug;11(8):1274-7.
Abstract Link: http://www.medifocus.com/abstracts.php?gid=NR015&ID=20704676

50.

Vasomotor disturbances in complex regional pain syndrome--a review.

Author: Wasner G
Institution: Department of Neurology, Division of Neurological Pain Research and
                   Therapy, University Clinic of Schleswig-Holstein, Kiel, Germany.
                   g.wasner@neurologie.uni-kiel.de
Journal: Pain Med. 2010 Aug;11(8):1267-73.
Abstract Link: http://www.medifocus.com/abstracts.php?gid=NR015&ID=20704675

51.

Fibromyalgia and the complex regional pain syndrome: similarities in pathophysiology and treatment.

Author: Wurtman RJ
Institution: Massachusetts Institute of Technology, Cambridge, MA 02139, USA.
                   dick@mit.edu
Journal: Metabolism. 2010 Oct;59 Suppl 1:S37-40.
Abstract Link: http://www.medifocus.com/abstracts.php?gid=NR015&ID=20837192

Go to http://www.medifocus.com/links/NR015/0314 for direct online access to the above Abstract Links.

52.

Is there an association between psychological factors and the Complex Regional Pain Syndrome type 1 (CRPS1) in adults? A systematic review.

Authors: Beerthuizen A; van 't Spijker A; Huygen FJ; Klein J; de Wit R
Institution: Department of Medical Psychology and Psychotherapy, Erasmus MC, Rotterdam, The Netherlands. a.beerthuizen@erasmusmc.nl
Journal: Pain. 2009 Sep;145(1-2):52-9. Epub 2009 Jul 1.
Abstract Link: http://www.medifocus.com/abstracts.php?gid=NR015&ID=19573987

53.

Pain: Do ACE inhibitors exacerbate complex regional pain syndrome?

Authors: Borsook D; Sava S
Institution: P.A.I.N. group, Department of Psychiatry, McLean Hospital, Belmont, MA, USA.
Journal: Nat Rev Neurol. 2009 Jun;5(6):306-8.
Abstract Link: http://www.medifocus.com/abstracts.php?gid=NR015&ID=19498433

54.

Current understandings on complex regional pain syndrome.

Authors: de Mos M; Sturkenboom MC; Huygen FJ
Institution: Erasmus University Medical Center, Pharmaco-epidemiology Unit, Departments of Medical Informatics and Epidemiology & Biostatistics, Rotterdam, The Netherlands. m.vrolijk-demos@erasmusmc.nl
Journal: Pain Pract. 2009 Mar-Apr;9(2):86-99. Epub 2008 Feb 9.
Abstract Link: http://www.medifocus.com/abstracts.php?gid=NR015&ID=19215592

Go to http://www.medifocus.com/links/NR015/0314 for direct online access to the above Abstract Links.

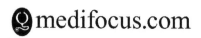

55.

Systematic review of the effectiveness of mirror therapy in upper extremity function.

Authors:	Ezendam D; Bongers RM; Jannink MJ
Institution:	Center for Human Movement Sciences, University of Groningen, University Medical Center Groningen, Groningen, The Netherlands.
Journal:	Disabil Rehabil. 2009 May 20:1-15.
Abstract Link:	http://www.medifocus.com/abstracts.php?gid=NR015&ID=19479545

56.

Systematic review of the effectiveness of mirror therapy in upper extremity function.

Authors:	Ezendam D; Bongers RM; Jannink MJ
Institution:	Center for Human Movement Sciences, University of Groningen, University Medical Center Groningen, Groningen, The Netherlands.
Journal:	Disabil Rehabil. 2009;31(26):2135-49.
Abstract Link:	http://www.medifocus.com/abstracts.php?gid=NR015&ID=19903124

57.

Spinal cord stimulation: principles of past, present and future practice: a review.

Authors:	Kunnumpurath S; Srinivasagopalan R; Vadivelu N
Institution:	St George's School of Anaesthesia, Tooting, London, UK. dreeku@doctors.org.uk
Journal:	J Clin Monit Comput. 2009 Oct;23(5):333-9.
Abstract Link:	http://www.medifocus.com/abstracts.php?gid=NR015&ID=19728120

Go to http://www.medifocus.com/links/NR015/0314 for direct online access to the above Abstract Links.

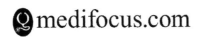

58.

Algodystrophy Treated with Needle-Free Electroacupuncture and Raw Chinese Herbal Decoction: A Case Report and Review of Literature.

Author:	Miao EY
Institution:	M. Modern TCM Clinic , Melbourne, Victoria, Australia .
Journal:	J Altern Complement Med. 2009 Sep 28.
Abstract Link:	http://www.medifocus.com/abstracts.php?gid=NR015&ID=19785531

59.

Is reflex sympathetic dystrophy/complex regional pain syndrome type I a small-fiber neuropathy?

Authors:	Oaklander AL; Fields HL
Institution:	Department of Neurology, Massachusetts General Hospital, Harvard Medical School, Boston, MA 02114, USA. aoaklander@partners.org
Journal:	Ann Neurol. 2009 Jun;65(6):629-38.
Abstract Link:	http://www.medifocus.com/abstracts.php?gid=NR015&ID=19557864

60.

The use of visual feedback, in particular mirror visual feedback, in restoring brain function.

Authors:	Ramachandran VS; Altschuler EL
Institution:	Center for Brain and Cognition, University of California, San Diego, 9500 Gilman Drive, 0109, La Jolla, California 92093-0109, USA. vramacha@ucsd.edu
Journal:	Brain. 2009 Jul;132(Pt 7):1693-710. Epub 2009 Jun 8.
Abstract Link:	http://www.medifocus.com/abstracts.php?gid=NR015&ID=19506071

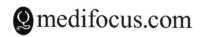

General Interest Articles

61.

Complex regional pain syndrome: practical diagnostic and treatment guidelines, 4th edition.

Authors:	Harden RN; Oaklander AL; Burton AW; Perez RS; Richardson K; Swan M; Barthel J; Costa B; Graciosa JR; Bruehl S
Institution:	Center for Pain Studies, Rehabilitation Institute of Chicago, Illinois 60611, USA. nharden@ric.org
Journal:	Pain Med. 2013 Feb;14(2):180-229. doi: 10.1111/pme.12033. Epub 2013 Jan 17.
Abstract Link:	http://www.medifocus.com/abstracts.php?gid=NR015&ID=23331950

62.

Children and adolescents with complex regional pain syndrome: more psychologically distressed than other children in pain?

Authors:	Logan DE; Williams SE; Carullo VP; Claar RL; Bruehl S; Berde CB
Institution:	Division of Pain Medicine, Department of Anesthesiology, Periperative and Pain Medicine, Children's Hospital, Boston, Massachusetts 02115, USA. deridre.logan@childrens.harvard.edu
Journal:	Pain Res Manag. 2013 Mar-Apr;18(2):87-93.
Abstract Link:	http://www.medifocus.com/abstracts.php?gid=NR015&ID=23662291

63.

The role of pain coping and kinesiophobia in patients with complex regional pain syndrome type 1 of the legs.

Authors:	Marinus J; Perez RS; van Eijs F; van Gestel MA; Geurts JW; Huygen FJ; Bauer MC; van Hilten JJ
Institution:	Department of Neurology, Leiden University Medical Center, The Netherlands. j.marinus@lumc.nl
Journal:	Clin J Pain. 2013 Jul;29(7):563-9. doi: 10.1097/AJP.0b013e31826f9a8a.
Abstract Link:	http://www.medifocus.com/abstracts.php?gid=NR015&ID=23739533

Go to http://www.medifocus.com/links/NR015/0314 for direct online access to the above Abstract Links.

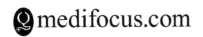

64.

Successive multisite peripheral nerve catheters for treatment of complex regional pain syndrome type I.

Authors: Martin DP; Bhalla T; Rehman S; Tobias JD
Institution: Department of aAnesthesiology and Pain Medicine, Nationwide Children's Hospital and the Ohio State University, Columbus, Ohio 43205, USA.
Journal: Pediatrics. 2013 Jan;131(1):e323-6. doi: 10.1542/peds.2011-3779. Epub 2012 Dec 10.
Abstract Link: http://www.medifocus.com/abstracts.php?gid=NR015&ID=23230070

65.

Complex regional pain syndrome following lateral lumbar interbody fusion: case report.

Authors: Morr S; Kanter AS
Institution: Department of Neurological Surgery, University of Pittsburgh Medical Center, Pittsburgh, Pennsylvania.
Journal: J Neurosurg Spine. 2013 Oct;19(4):502-6. doi: 10.3171/2013.7.SPINE12352. Epub 2013 Aug 16.
Abstract Link: http://www.medifocus.com/abstracts.php?gid=NR015&ID=23952321

66.

Changes resembling complex regional pain syndrome following surgery and immobilization.

Authors: Pepper A; Li W; Kingery WS; Angst MS; Curtin CM; Clark JD
Institution: Department of Anesthesia, Stanford University, Palo Alto, California, USA.
Journal: J Pain. 2013 May;14(5):516-24. doi: 10.1016/j.jpain.2013.01.004. Epub 2013 Feb 28.
Abstract Link: http://www.medifocus.com/abstracts.php?gid=NR015&ID=23453564

Go to http://www.medifocus.com/links/NR015/0314 for direct online access to the above Abstract Links.

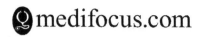

67.

Coping with chronic complex regional pain syndrome: advice from patients for patients.

Authors:	Rodham K; McCabe C; Pilkington M; Regan L
Institution:	Department of Psychology, University of Bath, Bath, UK. psskr@bath.ac.uk
Journal:	Chronic Illn. 2013 Mar;9(1):29-42. doi: 10.1177/1742395312450178. Epub 2012 Jun 1.
Abstract Link:	http://www.medifocus.com/abstracts.php?gid=NR015&ID=22659350

68.

Complex regional pain syndrome: observations on diagnosis, treatment and definition of a new subgroup.

Authors:	Zyluk A; Puchalski P
Institution:	Department of General and Hand Surgery, Pomeranian Medical University in Szczecin, Szczecin, Poland. azyluk@hotmail.com
Journal:	J Hand Surg Eur Vol. 2013 Jul;38(6):599-606. doi: 10.1177/1753193412469143. Epub 2012 Dec 6.
Abstract Link:	http://www.medifocus.com/abstracts.php?gid=NR015&ID=23221182

69.

Complex regional pain syndrome following protracted labour*.

Authors:	Butchart AG; Mathews M; Surendran A
Institution:	Department of Anaesthesia, Norfolk & Norwich University Hospital, Norwich, Norfolk, UK. angusbutchart@doctors.org.uk
Journal:	Anaesthesia. 2012 Nov;67(11):1272-4. doi: 10.1111/j.1365-2044.2012.07301.x. Epub 2012 Aug 7.
Abstract Link:	http://www.medifocus.com/abstracts.php?gid=NR015&ID=22881282

Go to http://www.medifocus.com/links/NR015/0314 for direct online access to the above Abstract Links.

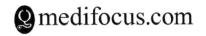

70.

Anxious personality is a risk factor for developing complex regional pain syndrome type I.

Authors: Dilek B; Yemez B; Kizil R; Kartal E; Gulbahar S; Sari O; Akalin E
Institution: Department of Physical Medicine and Rehabilitation, Dokuz Eylul University Faculty of Medicine, Inciralti, Izmir, Turkey. banudilek1979@gmail.com
Journal: Rheumatol Int. 2012 Apr;32(4):915-20. Epub 2011 Jan 15.
Abstract Link: http://www.medifocus.com/abstracts.php?gid=NR015&ID=21240501

71.

Complex regional pain syndrome of the pediatric lower extremity: a retrospective review.

Authors: Harris EJ; Schimka KE; Carlson RM
Institution: Section of Podiatry, Department of Orthopedic Surgery, Loyola University Medical Center, Maywood, IL, USA.
Journal: J Am Podiatr Med Assoc. 2012 Mar-Apr;102(2):99-104.
Abstract Link: http://www.medifocus.com/abstracts.php?gid=NR015&ID=22461266

72.

Chinese scalp acupuncture relieves pain and restores function in complex regional pain syndrome.

Author: Hommer DH
Institution: Physical Medicine and Rehabilitation Service, Department of Orthopedics and Rehabilitation, Brooke Army Medical Center, 3551 Roger Brooke Drive, Fort Sam Houston, TX 78234, USA.
Journal: Mil Med. 2012 Oct;177(10):1231-4.
Abstract Link: http://www.medifocus.com/abstracts.php?gid=NR015&ID=23113454

Go to http://www.medifocus.com/links/NR015/0314 for direct online access to the above Abstract Links.

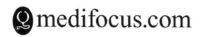

73.

Skin biopsy in complex regional pain syndrome: case series and literature review.

Authors: Kharkar S; Venkatesh YS; Grothusen JR; Rojas L; Schwartzman RJ
Institution: Department of Neurology, Drexel University College of Medicine, Philadelphia, PA, USA.
Journal: Pain Physician. 2012 May-Jun;15(3):255-66.
Abstract Link: http://www.medifocus.com/abstracts.php?gid=NR015&ID=22622910

74.

Cognitive correlates of "neglect-like syndrome" in patients with complex regional pain syndrome.

Authors: Kolb L; Lang C; Seifert F; Maihofner C
Institution: Department of Neurology, University Hospital Erlangen, Erlangen, Germany.
Journal: Pain. 2012 May;153(5):1063-73. Epub 2012 Mar 16.
Abstract Link: http://www.medifocus.com/abstracts.php?gid=NR015&ID=22424691

75.

Modified graded motor imagery for complex regional pain syndrome type 1 of the upper extremity in the acute phase: a patient series.

Authors: Lagueux E; Charest J; Lefrancois-Caron E; Mauger ME; Mercier E; Savard K; Tousignant-Laflamme Y
Institution: Faculty of Medicine and Health Sciences, University of Sherbrooke, Quebec, Canada.
Journal: Int J Rehabil Res. 2012 Jun;35(2):138-45.
Abstract Link: http://www.medifocus.com/abstracts.php?gid=NR015&ID=22436440

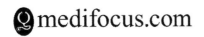

76.

Perceptions of the painful body: the relationship between body perception disturbance, pain and tactile discrimination in complex regional pain syndrome.

Authors:	Lewis JS; Schweinhardt P
Institution:	Faculty of Dentistry, McGill University, Montreal, Canada. jenslewis@hotmail.com
Journal:	Eur J Pain. 2012 Oct;16(9):1320-30. doi: 10.1002/j.1532-2149.2012.00120.x. Epub 2012 Mar 9.
Abstract Link:	http://www.medifocus.com/abstracts.php?gid=NR015&ID=22407949

77.

Hypothalamic-pituitary-adrenal axis function in patients with complex regional pain syndrome type 1.

Authors:	Park JY; Ahn RS
Institution:	Department of Anesthesiology and Pain Medicine, The Armed Forces Capital Hospital, Seoul, Republic of Korea.
Journal:	Psychoneuroendocrinology. 2012 Sep;37(9):1557-68. doi: 10.1016/j.psyneuen.2012.02.016. Epub 2012 Mar 24.
Abstract Link:	http://www.medifocus.com/abstracts.php?gid=NR015&ID=22445364

78.

Impaired oxygen utilization in skeletal muscle of CRPS I patients.

Authors:	Tan EC; Ter Laak HJ; Hopman MT; van Goor H; Goris RJ
Institution:	Department of Surgery, Radboud University Nijmegen Medical Centre, Nijmegen, The Netherlands. E.Tan@chir.umcn.nl
Journal:	J Surg Res. 2012 Mar;173(1):145-52. Epub 2010 Sep 16.
Abstract Link:	http://www.medifocus.com/abstracts.php?gid=NR015&ID=20934715

Go to http://www.medifocus.com/links/NR015/0314 for direct online access to the above Abstract Links.

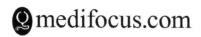
medifocus.com

79.

Poor prognostic factors in complex regional pain syndrome 1: a Delphi survey.

Authors: Brunner F; Nauer M; Bachmann LM

Institution: Department of Physical Medicine and Rheumatology, Balgrist University Hospital, Forchstrasse 340, CH-8008 Zurich, Switzerland. florian.brunner@balgrist.ch

Journal: J Rehabil Med. 2011 Sep;43(9):783-6.
Abstract Link: http://www.medifocus.com/abstracts.php?gid=NR015&ID=21874213

80.

Complex Regional Pain Syndrome: What's in a Name?

Author: Coderre TJ

Institution: Department of Anesthesia and Alan Edward Centre for Research on Pain, McGill University, and McGill University Health Centre Research Institute, Montreal, Quebec.

Journal: J Pain. 2011 Jan;12(1):2-12. Epub 2010 Jul 15.
Abstract Link: http://www.medifocus.com/abstracts.php?gid=NR015&ID=20634146

81.

Emotional and neuropsychological profiles of children with complex regional pain syndrome type-I in an inpatient rehabilitation setting.

Authors: Cruz N; O'Reilly J; Slomine BS; Salorio CF

Institution: Department of Psychology, St. Louis Children's Hospital, One Children's Place, St. Louis, MO 63118, USA. nxc2032@bjc.org

Journal: Clin J Pain. 2011 Jan;27(1):27-34.
Abstract Link: http://www.medifocus.com/abstracts.php?gid=NR015&ID=20842016

Go to http://www.medifocus.com/links/NR015/0314 for direct online access to the above Abstract Links.

82.

Distribution of signs and symptoms of complex regional pain syndrome type I in patients meeting the diagnostic criteria of the International Association for the Study of Pain.

Authors: de Boer RD; Marinus J; van Hilten JJ; Huygen FJ; van Eijs F; van Kleef M; Bauer MC; van Gestel M; Zuurmond WW; Perez RS

Institution: Department of Anesthesiology, VU University Medical Center, Amsterdam, The Netherlands. rdh.deboer@vumc.nl

Journal: Eur J Pain. 2011 Sep;15(8):830.e1-8. Epub 2011 Feb 22.

Abstract Link: http://www.medifocus.com/abstracts.php?gid=NR015&ID=21334934

83.

Pain-related fear, perceived harmfulness of activities, and functional limitations in complex regional pain syndrome type I.

Authors: de Jong JR; Vlaeyen JW; de Gelder JM; Patijn J

Institution: Department of Rehabilitation, University Hospital Maastricht, Maastricht, The Netherlands. jeroen.dejong@mumc.nl

Journal: J Pain. 2011 Dec;12(12):1209-18. Epub 2011 Oct 26.

Abstract Link: http://www.medifocus.com/abstracts.php?gid=NR015&ID=22033012

84.

Complex interaction of sensory and motor signs and symptoms in chronic CRPS.

Authors: Huge V; Lauchart M; Magerl W; Beyer A; Moehnle P; Kaufhold W; Schelling G; Azad SC

Institution: Department of Anaesthesiology, Ludwig-Maximilians-Universitat Munchen, Munich, Germany. vhuge@med.uni-muenchen.de

Journal: PLoS One. 2011 Apr 29;6(4):e18775.

Abstract Link: http://www.medifocus.com/abstracts.php?gid=NR015&ID=21559525

Go to http://www.medifocus.com/links/NR015/0314 for direct online access to the above Abstract Links.

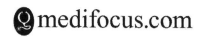

85.

Early aggressive treatment improves prognosis in complex regional pain syndrome.

Authors: Lee J; Nandi P

Institution: Pain Management Centre, National Hospital for Neurology & Neurosurgery, Queen Square, London.

Journal: Practitioner. 2011 Jan;255(1736):23-6, 3.

Abstract Link: http://www.medifocus.com/abstracts.php?gid=NR015&ID=21370711

86.

Turning the nightmare of complex regional pain syndrome into a time of healing, renewal, and hope.

Authors: Montana C; Kautz DD

Institution: Midwestern University, Glendale, AZ, USA.

Journal: Medsurg Nurs. 2011 May-Jun;20(3):139-42.

Abstract Link: http://www.medifocus.com/abstracts.php?gid=NR015&ID=21786490

87.

Thermal hypesthesia in patients with complex regional pain syndrome related dystonia.

Authors: Munts AG; van Rijn MA; Geraedts EJ; van Hilten JJ; van Dijk JG; Marinus J

Institution: Department of Neurology, Leiden University Medical Center, P.O. Box 9600, 2300 RC, Leiden, The Netherlands.

Journal: J Neural Transm. 2011 Apr;118(4):599-603. Epub 2010 Dec 29.

Abstract Link: http://www.medifocus.com/abstracts.php?gid=NR015&ID=21190049

Go to http://www.medifocus.com/links/NR015/0314 for direct online access to the above Abstract Links.

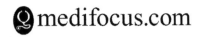

88.

Syncope in complex regional pain syndrome.

Authors:	Smith JA; Karalis DG; Rosso AL; Grothusen JR; Hessen SE; Schwartzman RJ
Institution:	Department of Cardiology, Drexel University College of Medicine, Philadelphia, Pennsylvania, USA. doctorjay21074@yahoo.com
Journal:	Clin Cardiol. 2011 Apr;34(4):222-5. doi: 10.1002/clc.20879.
Abstract Link:	http://www.medifocus.com/abstracts.php?gid=NR015&ID=21462216

89.

Integrative approach focusing on acupuncture in the treatment of chronic complex regional pain syndrome.

Authors:	Sprague M; Chang JC
Institution:	Coastal Carolina Neuropsychiatric Center, Jacksonville, NC, USA.
Journal:	J Altern Complement Med. 2011 Jan;17(1):67-70. Epub 2011 Jan 5.
Abstract Link:	http://www.medifocus.com/abstracts.php?gid=NR015&ID=21208130

90.

Safety of "pain exposure" physical therapy in patients with complex regional pain syndrome type 1.

Authors:	van de Meent H; Oerlemans M; Bruggeman A; Klomp F; van Dongen R; Oostendorp R; Frolke JP
Institution:	Department of Rehabilitation, Nijmegen Centre of Evidence Based Practice, Radboud University Nijmegen Medical Centre, Nijmegen, The Netherlands. h.vandemeent@reval.umcn.nl
Journal:	Pain. 2011 Jun;152(6):1431-8. Epub 2011 Apr 6.
Abstract Link:	http://www.medifocus.com/abstracts.php?gid=NR015&ID=21474244

Go to http://www.medifocus.com/links/NR015/0314 for direct online access to the above Abstract Links.

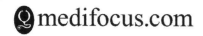
91.

Evidence-based interventional pain medicine according to clinical diagnoses. 16. Complex regional pain syndrome.

Authors:	van Eijs F; Stanton-Hicks M; Van Zundert J; Faber CG; Lubenow TR; Mekhail N; van Kleef M; Huygen F
Institution:	Department of Anesthesiology and Pain Therapy, St. Elisabeth Hospital, Tilburg, The Netherlands.
Journal:	Pain Pract. 2011 Jan-Feb;11(1):70-87. doi: 10.1111/j.1533-2500.2010.00388.x. Epub 2010 Aug 27.
Abstract Link:	http://www.medifocus.com/abstracts.php?gid=NR015&ID=20807353

92.

Spreading of complex regional pain syndrome: not a random process.

Authors:	van Rijn MA; Marinus J; Putter H; Bosselaar SR; Moseley GL; van Hilten JJ
Institution:	Department of Neurology (K5Q), Leiden University Medical Center, P.O. Box 9600, 2300 RC, Leiden, The Netherlands. m.a.van_rijn@lumc.nl
Journal:	J Neural Transm. 2011 Sep;118(9):1301-9. Epub 2011 Feb 18.
Abstract Link:	http://www.medifocus.com/abstracts.php?gid=NR015&ID=21331457

93.

Biopsychosocial complexity is correlated with psychiatric comorbidity but not with perceived pain in complex regional pain syndrome type 1 (algodystrophy) of the knee.

Authors:	Vouilloz A; Deriaz O; Rivier G; Gobelet C; Luthi F
Institution:	Clinique Romande de Readaptation SuvaCare, avenue Grand-Champsec 90, 1951 Sion, Switzerland. aurelie.vouilloz@crr-suva.ch
Journal:	Joint Bone Spine. 2011 Mar;78(2):194-9. Epub 2010 Sep 20.
Abstract Link:	http://www.medifocus.com/abstracts.php?gid=NR015&ID=20851028

Go to http://www.medifocus.com/links/NR015/0314 for direct online access to the above Abstract Links.

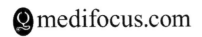

94.

The first scintigraphic detection of tumor necrosis factor-alpha in patients with complex regional pain syndrome type 1.

Authors: Bernateck M; Karst M; Gratz KF; Meyer GJ; Fischer MJ; Knapp WH; Koppert W; Brunkhorst T

Institution: Department of Anesthesiology, Pain Clinic, Hannover Medical School, Carl-Neuberg-Str. 1, Hannover 30625, Germany. bernateck.michael@mh-hannover.de

Journal: Anesth Analg. 2010 Jan;110(1):211-5. Epub 2009 Nov 12.

Abstract Link: http://www.medifocus.com/abstracts.php?gid=NR015&ID=19910617

95.

Disease-related knowledge of patients with chronic regional pain syndrome.

Authors: Brunner F; Gymesi A; Kissling R; Bachmann LM

Institution: Department of Physical Medicine and Rheumatology, Balgrist University Hospital, Forchstrasse 340, 8008 Zurich, Switzerland. florian.brunner@balgrist.ch

Journal: J Rehabil Med. 2010 May;42(5):458-62.

Abstract Link: http://www.medifocus.com/abstracts.php?gid=NR015&ID=20544157

96.

Poststroke complex regional pain syndrome.

Author: Chae J

Institution: Department of Physical Medicine and Rehabilitation, Case Western Reserve University, Cleveland, Ohio, USA.

Journal: Top Stroke Rehabil. 2010 May-Jun;17(3):151-62.

Abstract Link: http://www.medifocus.com/abstracts.php?gid=NR015&ID=20797958

Go to http://www.medifocus.com/links/NR015/0314 for direct online access to the above Abstract Links.

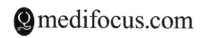
97.

Spontaneous onset of complex regional pain syndrome.

Authors: de Rooij AM; Perez RS; Huygen FJ; Eijs FV; Kleef MV; Bauer MC;
                      van Hilten JJ; Marinus J; van Eijs F; van Kleef M
Institution: Department of Neurology, Leiden University Medical Center, Leiden,
                      The Netherlands.
Journal: Eur J Pain. 2010 May;14(5):510-3. Epub 2009 Sep 29.
Abstract Link: http://www.medifocus.com/abstracts.php?gid=NR015&ID=19793666

98.

Lower extremity complex regional pain syndrome: long-term outcome after surgical treatment of peripheral pain generators.

Authors: Dellon L; Andonian E; Rosson GD
Institution: Johns Hopkins University, Baltimore, MD, USA.
                      ALDellon@Dellon.com
Journal: J Foot Ankle Surg. 2010 Jan-Feb;49(1):33-6.
Abstract Link: http://www.medifocus.com/abstracts.php?gid=NR015&ID=20123284

99.

Complex regional pain syndrome: a vitamin K dependent entity?

Authors: Ediz L; Hiz O; Meral I; Alpayci M
Institution: Yuzuncu Yil University Medical Faculty, Physical Medicine and
                      Rehabilitation Department, 65100 Van, Turkey.
                      leventediz@gmail.com
Journal: Med Hypotheses. 2010 Sep;75(3):319-23. Epub 2010 Apr 7.
Abstract Link: http://www.medifocus.com/abstracts.php?gid=NR015&ID=20378261

Go to http://www.medifocus.com/links/NR015/0314 for direct online access to the above Abstract Links.

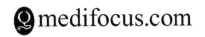

100.

Validation of proposed diagnostic criteria (the "Budapest Criteria") for Complex Regional Pain Syndrome.

Authors:	Harden RN; Bruehl S; Perez RS; Birklein F; Marinus J; Maihofner C; Lubenow T; Buvanendran A; Mackey S; Graciosa J; Mogilevski M; Ramsden C; Chont M; Vatine JJ
Institution:	Rehabilitation Institute of Chicago, Chicago, IL 60611, USA. nharden@ric.org
Journal:	Pain. 2010 Aug;150(2):268-74. Epub 2010 May 20.
Abstract Link:	http://www.medifocus.com/abstracts.php?gid=NR015&ID=20493633

101.

Objectification of the diagnostic criteria for CRPS.

Author:	Harden RN
Institution:	Rehabilitation Institute of Chicago, Northwestern University, Chicago, Illinois 60611, USA.
Journal:	Pain Med. 2010 Aug;11(8):1212-5.
Abstract Link:	http://www.medifocus.com/abstracts.php?gid=NR015&ID=20704669

102.

Complex regional pain syndrome/reflex sympathetic dystrophy.

Authors:	Jakubowicz B; Aner M
Institution:	Pain Medicine at Harvard Medical School, Beth Israel Deaconess Medical Center, Boston, Massachusetts 07503, USA. bmjakubowicz@gmail.com
Journal:	J Pain Palliat Care Pharmacother. 2010 Jun;24(2):160-1.
Abstract Link:	http://www.medifocus.com/abstracts.php?gid=NR015&ID=20504141

Go to http://www.medifocus.com/links/NR015/0314 for direct online access to the above Abstract Links.

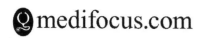

103.

The fascination of complex regional pain syndrome.

Author: Janig W

Institution: Physiologisches Institut, Christian-Albrechts-Universitat zu Kiel, Kiel, Germany. w.janig@physiologie.uni-kiel.de

Journal: Exp Neurol. 2010 Jan;221(1):1-4. Epub 2009 Sep 30.

Abstract Link: http://www.medifocus.com/abstracts.php?gid=NR015&ID=19799902

104.

Wherever is my arm? Impaired upper limb position accuracy in complex regional pain syndrome.

Authors: Lewis JS; Kersten P; McPherson KM; Taylor GJ; Harris N; McCabe CS; Blake DR

Institution: McGill University, Montreal, Canada. jenslewis@hotmail.com

Journal: Pain. 2010 Jun;149(3):463-9. Epub 2010 Apr 10.

Abstract Link: http://www.medifocus.com/abstracts.php?gid=NR015&ID=20385441

105.

Neuropsychological deficits associated with Complex Regional Pain Syndrome.

Authors: Libon DJ; Schwartzman RJ; Eppig J; Wambach D; Brahin E; Lee Peterlin B; Alexander G; Kalanuria A

Institution: Department of Neurology, Drexel University, College of Medicine, Philadelphia, PA 19102, USA. dlibon@Drexelmed.edu

Journal: J Int Neuropsychol Soc. 2010 May;16(3):566-73. Epub 2010 Mar 19.

Abstract Link: http://www.medifocus.com/abstracts.php?gid=NR015&ID=20298641

Go to http://www.medifocus.com/links/NR015/0314 for direct online access to the above Abstract Links.

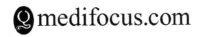

106.

Neuropathic pain syndrome displayed by malingerers.

Authors: Ochoa JL; Verdugo RJ

Institution: The Oregon Nerve Center, Good Samaritan Medical Center, 1040 NW
22nd Ave., Suite 600, Portland, OR 97210, USA.
jochoa@nervesense.net

Journal: J Neuropsychiatry Clin Neurosci. 2010 Summer;22(3):278-86.

Abstract Link: http://www.medifocus.com/abstracts.php?gid=NR015&ID=20686134

107.

Evidence based guidelines for complex regional pain syndrome type 1.

Authors: Perez RS; Zollinger PE; Dijkstra PU; Thomassen-Hilgersom IL;
Zuurmond WW; Rosenbrand KC; Geertzen JH

Institution: VU University Medical Center, Department of Anaesthesiology,
Amsterdam, the Netherlands. rsgm.perez@vumc.nl

Journal: BMC Neurol. 2010 Mar 31;10:20.

Abstract Link: http://www.medifocus.com/abstracts.php?gid=NR015&ID=20356382

108.

Do omega-6 and trans fatty acids play a role in complex regional pain syndrome? A pilot study.

Authors: Ramsden C; Gagnon C; Graciosa J; Faurot K; David R; Bralley JA;
Harden RN

Institution: Rehabilitation Institute of Chicago, Department of Physical Medicine
and Rehabilitation, Northwestern University Feinberg School of
Medicine, Chicago, Illinois, USA. chris.ramsden@nih.gov

Journal: Pain Med. 2010 Jul;11(7):1115-25. Epub 2010 Jun 8.

Abstract Link: http://www.medifocus.com/abstracts.php?gid=NR015&ID=20545870

Go to http://www.medifocus.com/links/NR015/0314 for direct online access to the above Abstract Links.

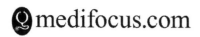
109.

Nonimmersive virtual reality mirror visual feedback therapy and its application for the treatment of complex regional pain syndrome: an open-label pilot study.

Authors:	Sato K; Fukumori S; Matsusaki T; Maruo T; Ishikawa S; Nishie H; Takata K; Mizuhara H; Mizobuchi S; Nakatsuka H; Matsumi M; Gofuku A; Yokoyama M; Morita K
Institution:	Department of Anesthesiology and Resuscitology, Okayama University Graduate School of Medicine and Dentistry, Okayama City, Okayama Prefecture, 700-8551, Japan. tento@cc.okayama-u.ac.jp
Journal:	Pain Med. 2010 Apr;11(4):622-9. Epub 2010 Mar 1.
Abstract Link:	http://www.medifocus.com/abstracts.php?gid=NR015&ID=20202141

110.

Familial occurrence of complex regional pain syndrome.

Authors:	Shirani P; Jawaid A; Moretti P; Lahijani E; Salamone AR; Schulz PE; Edmondson EA
Institution:	Department of Neurology, Baylor College of Medicine, Houston, Texas, USA.
Journal:	Can J Neurol Sci. 2010 May;37(3):389-94.
Abstract Link:	http://www.medifocus.com/abstracts.php?gid=NR015&ID=20481275

111.

Diagnostic criteria in patients with complex regional pain syndrome assessed in an out-patient clinic.

Authors:	Van Bodegraven Hof EA; Groeneweg GJ; Wesseldijk F; Huygen FJ; Zijlstra FJ
Institution:	Department of Anesthesiology, Pain Treatment Centre, Erasmus MC, Rotterdam, the Netherlands.
Journal:	Acta Anaesthesiol Scand. 2010 Aug;54(7):894-9. Epub 2010 May 27.
Abstract Link:	http://www.medifocus.com/abstracts.php?gid=NR015&ID=20528779

Go to http://www.medifocus.com/links/NR015/0314 for direct online access to the above Abstract Links.

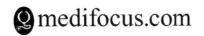

112.

Sympathetic dysfunction in long-term complex regional pain syndrome.

Authors: Vogel T; Gradl G; Ockert B; Pellengahr CS; Schurmann M
Institution: Department of Orthopedic Surgery, University of Bochum, Germany. t.vogel@klinikum-bochum.de
Journal: Clin J Pain. 2010 Feb;26(2):128-31.
Abstract Link: http://www.medifocus.com/abstracts.php?gid=NR015&ID=20090439

113.

Complex regional pain syndrome type 1. Some treatments assessed versus placebo, limited efficacy.

Author:
Journal: Prescrire Int. 2009 Dec;18(104):267-71.
Abstract Link: http://www.medifocus.com/abstracts.php?gid=NR015&ID=20027710

114.

Movement disorders associated with complex regional pain syndrome in children.

Authors: Agrawal SK; Rittey CD; Harrower NA; Goddard JM; Mordekar SR
Institution: Department of Paediatric Neurology, Sheffield Children's Hospital, Sheffield, UK.
Journal: Dev Med Child Neurol. 2009 Jul;51(7):557-62. Epub 2008 Nov 19.
Abstract Link: http://www.medifocus.com/abstracts.php?gid=NR015&ID=19018846

115.

Mirror therapy in complex regional pain syndrome type 1 of the upper limb in stroke patients.

Authors: Cacchio A; De Blasis E; De Blasis V; Santilli V; Spacca G
Institution: Department of Physical Medicine and Rehabilitation, "San Salvatore" Hospital of L'Aquila, L'Aquila, Italy,angelo.cacchio@tin.it.
Journal: Neurorehabil Neural Repair. 2009 Oct;23(8):792-9. Epub 2009 May 22.
Abstract Link: http://www.medifocus.com/abstracts.php?gid=NR015&ID=19465507

Go to http://www.medifocus.com/links/NR015/0314 for direct online access to the above Abstract Links.

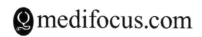

116.

Does prolonged skin temperature measurement improve the diagnosis of complex regional pain syndrome?

Authors: Cohen SP; Raja SN
Institution: Division of Pain Medicine, Department of Anesthesiology and Critical
                   Care Medicine at Johns Hopkins University School of Medicine,
                   Baltimore, MD 21287, USA.
Journal: Nat Clin Pract Neurol. 2009 Jan;5(1):14-5.
Abstract Link: http://www.medifocus.com/abstracts.php?gid=NR015&ID=19129786

117.

Does evidence support physiotherapy management of adult Complex Regional Pain Syndrome Type One? A systematic review.

Authors: Daly AE; Bialocerkowski AE
Institution: Department of Physiotherapy, Austin Hospital, Heidelberg 3084,
                   Victoria, Australia. anne.daly@austin.org.au
Journal: Eur J Pain. 2009 Apr;13(4):339-53. Epub 2008 Jul 10.
Abstract Link: http://www.medifocus.com/abstracts.php?gid=NR015&ID=18619873

118.

Estrogens and the risk of complex regional pain syndrome (CRPS).

Authors: de Mos M; Huygen FJ; Stricker BH; Dieleman JP; Sturkenboom MC
Institution: Pharmaco-Epidemiology Unit, Department of Medical Informatics and
                   Epidemiology & Biostatistics, Erasmus University Medical Center,
                   Rotterdam, The Netherlands. m.vrolijk-demos@erasmusmc.nl
Journal: Pharmacoepidemiol Drug Saf. 2009 Jan;18(1):44-52.
Abstract Link: http://www.medifocus.com/abstracts.php?gid=NR015&ID=19111016

Go to http://www.medifocus.com/links/NR015/0314 for direct online access to the above Abstract Links.

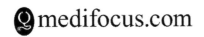

119.

The association between ACE inhibitors and the complex regional pain syndrome: Suggestions for a neuro-inflammatory pathogenesis of CRPS.

Authors: de Mos M; Huygen FJ; Stricker BH; Dieleman JP; Sturkenboom MC

Institution: Erasmus University Medical Center, Pharmaco-epidemiology Unit, Department of Medical Informatics and Epidemiology, Rotterdam, The Netherlands. m.vrolijk-demos@erasmusmc.nl

Journal: Pain. 2009 Apr;142(3):218-24. Epub 2009 Feb 4.

Abstract Link: http://www.medifocus.com/abstracts.php?gid=NR015&ID=19195784

120.

Outcome of the complex regional pain syndrome.

Authors: de Mos M; Huygen FJ; van der Hoeven-Borgman M; Dieleman JP; Ch Stricker BH; Sturkenboom MC

Institution: Departments of Medical Informatics and Epidemiology and Biostatistics, Erasmus University Medical Center, Rotterdam, The Netherlands. m.vrolijk-demos@erasmusmc.nl

Journal: Clin J Pain. 2009 Sep;25(7):590-7.

Abstract Link: http://www.medifocus.com/abstracts.php?gid=NR015&ID=19692800

121.

Familial occurrence of complex regional pain syndrome.

Authors: de Rooij AM; de Mos M; Sturkenboom MC; Marinus J; van den Maagdenberg AM; van Hilten JJ

Institution: Department of Neurology, Leiden University Medical Center, Leiden, The Netherlands.

Journal: Eur J Pain. 2009 Feb;13(2):171-7. Epub 2008 Jun 2.

Abstract Link: http://www.medifocus.com/abstracts.php?gid=NR015&ID=18514555

Go to http://www.medifocus.com/links/NR015/0314 for direct online access to the above Abstract Links.

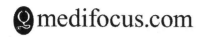
122.

Increased risk of complex regional pain syndrome in siblings of patients?

Authors:	de Rooij AM; de Mos M; van Hilten JJ; Sturkenboom MC; Gosso MF; van den Maagdenberg AM; Marinus J
Institution:	Department of Neurology, Leiden University Medical Center, Leiden, The Netherlands.
Journal:	J Pain. 2009 Dec;10(12):1250-5. Epub 2009 Oct 22.
Abstract Link:	http://www.medifocus.com/abstracts.php?gid=NR015&ID=19853528

123.

The efficacy of manual lymphatic drainage therapy in the management of limb edema secondary to reflex sympathetic dystrophy.

Authors:	Duman I; Ozdemir A; Tan AK; Dincer K
Institution:	Department of Physical Medicine and Rehabilitation, Gulhane Military Medical Academy, Etlik, 06018, Ankara, Turkey. iltekinduman@yahoo.com
Journal:	Rheumatol Int. 2009 May;29(7):759-63. Epub 2008 Nov 22.
Abstract Link:	http://www.medifocus.com/abstracts.php?gid=NR015&ID=19030864

124.

Warm and cold complex regional pain syndromes: differences beyond skin temperature?

Authors:	Eberle T; Doganci B; Kramer HH; Geber C; Fechir M; Magerl W; Birklein F
Institution:	Department of Neurology, Johannes Gutenberg University, Langenbeckstrasse 1, 55101 Mainz, Germany. eberlet@uni-mainz.de
Journal:	Neurology. 2009 Feb 10;72(6):505-12.
Abstract Link:	http://www.medifocus.com/abstracts.php?gid=NR015&ID=19204260

Go to http://www.medifocus.com/links/NR015/0314 for direct online access to the above Abstract Links.

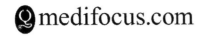

125.

Pain exposure physical therapy may be a safe and effective treatment for longstanding complex regional pain syndrome type 1: a case series.

Authors: Ek JW; van Gijn JC; Samwel H; van Egmond J; Klomp FP; van Dongen RT

Institution: Department of Rehabilitation Medicine, Bethesda Hospital, Hoogeveen.

Journal: Clin Rehabil. 2009 Dec;23(12):1059-66. Epub .

Abstract Link: http://www.medifocus.com/abstracts.php?gid=NR015&ID=19906762

126.

Regulation of peripheral blood flow in Complex Regional Pain Syndrome: clinical implication for symptomatic relief and pain management.

Authors: Groeneweg G; Huygen FJ; Coderre TJ; Zijlstra FJ

Institution: Department of Anesthesiology, Subdivision Pain Treatment Centre, Erasmus MC, Rotterdam, The Netherlands. j.groeneweg@erasmusmc.nl

Journal: BMC Musculoskelet Disord. 2009 Sep 23;10:116.

Abstract Link: http://www.medifocus.com/abstracts.php?gid=NR015&ID=19775468

127.

Practical management of complex regional pain syndrome.

Author: Hsu ES

Institution: Pain Management Center, Department of Anesthesiology, David Geffen School of Medicine, University of California, Los Angeles, LA, USA. ehsu@mednet.ucla.edu

Journal: Am J Ther. 2009 Mar-Apr;16(2):147-54.

Abstract Link: http://www.medifocus.com/abstracts.php?gid=NR015&ID=19300041

Go to http://www.medifocus.com/links/NR015/0314 for direct online access to the above Abstract Links.

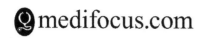

128.

Myopathy in CRPS-I: disuse or neurogenic?

Authors: Hulsman NM; Geertzen JH; Dijkstra PU; van den Dungen JJ; den Dunnen WF

Institution: Centre for Rehabilitation, University Medical Centre Groningen, University of Groningen, PO Box 30001, 9700 RB Groningen, The Netherlands. n.m.hulsman@rev.umcg.nl

Journal: Eur J Pain. 2009 Aug;13(7):731-6. Epub 2008 Oct 31.

Abstract Link: http://www.medifocus.com/abstracts.php?gid=NR015&ID=18976942

129.

The effect of tactile discrimination training is enhanced when patients watch the reflected image of their unaffected limb during training.

Authors: Moseley GL; Wiech K

Institution: Department of Physiology, Anatomy & Genetics, University of Oxford, Oxford, UK. lorimer.moseley@gmail.com

Journal: Pain. 2009 Aug;144(3):314-9. Epub 2009 Jun 6.

Abstract Link: http://www.medifocus.com/abstracts.php?gid=NR015&ID=19501965

130.

Migraine may be a risk factor for the development of complex regional pain syndrome.

Authors: Peterlin BL; Rosso AL; Nair S; Young WB; Schwartzman RJ

Institution: Department of Neurology, Drexel University College of Medicine, Philadelphia, PA, USA.

Journal: Cephalalgia. 2009 Jul 9.

Abstract Link: http://www.medifocus.com/abstracts.php?gid=NR015&ID=19614690

Go to http://www.medifocus.com/links/NR015/0314 for direct online access to the above Abstract Links.

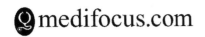

131.

Seeking support: An interpretative phenomenological analysis of an Internet message board for people with Complex Regional Pain Syndrome.

Authors:	Rodham K; McCabe C; Blake D
Institution:	Department of Psychology, University of Bath, UK. psskr@bath.ac.uk
Journal:	Psychol Health. 2009 Jul;24(6):619-34.
Abstract Link:	http://www.medifocus.com/abstracts.php?gid=NR015&ID=20205016

132.

Role of biphosphonates and lymphatic drainage type Leduc in the complex regional pain syndrome (shoulder-hand syndrome).

Authors:	Santamato A; Ranieri M; Panza F; Solfrizzi V; Frisardi V; Stolfa I; Megna M; Fiore P
Institution:	Department of Physical Medicine and Rehabilitation, University of Foggia, Foggia, Italy.
Journal:	Pain Med. 2009 Jan;10(1):179-85.
Abstract Link:	http://www.medifocus.com/abstracts.php?gid=NR015&ID=19222778

133.

The effect of sequel symptoms and signs of Complex Regional Pain Syndrome type 1 on upper extremity disability and quality of life.

Authors:	Savas S; Baloglu HH; Ay G; Cerci SS
Institution:	Department of Physical Medicine and Rehabilitation, Suleyman Demirel University Medical School, Isparta, Turkey. serpilsavas@yahoo.com
Journal:	Rheumatol Int. 2009 Mar;29(5):545-50. Epub 2008 Oct 25.
Abstract Link:	http://www.medifocus.com/abstracts.php?gid=NR015&ID=18953539

Go to http://www.medifocus.com/links/NR015/0314 for direct online access to the above Abstract Links.

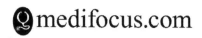
134.

The natural history of complex regional pain syndrome.

Authors: Schwartzman RJ; Erwin KL; Alexander GM
Institution: Department of Neurology, Drexel University College of Medicine, Philadelphia, PA 19102, USA. robert.schwartzman@drexelmed.edu
Journal: Clin J Pain. 2009 May;25(4):273-80.
Abstract Link: http://www.medifocus.com/abstracts.php?gid=NR015&ID=19590474

135.

A web-based cross-sectional epidemiological survey of complex regional pain syndrome.

Authors: Sharma A; Agarwal S; Broatch J; Raja SN
Institution: Department of Anesthesiology, College of Physicians & Surgeons of Columbia University, New York, NY, USA.
Journal: Reg Anesth Pain Med. 2009 Mar-Apr;34(2):110-5.
Abstract Link: http://www.medifocus.com/abstracts.php?gid=NR015&ID=19282709

136.

Cortical changes in complex regional pain syndrome (CRPS).

Authors: Swart CM; Stins JF; Beek PJ
Institution: Research Institute MOVE, Faculty of Human Movement Sciences, VU University Amsterdam, van der Boechorststraat 9, 1081 BT Amsterdam, The Netherlands.
Journal: Eur J Pain. 2009 Oct;13(9):902-7. Epub 2008 Dec 19.
Abstract Link: http://www.medifocus.com/abstracts.php?gid=NR015&ID=19101181

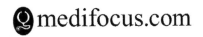
137.

Quality of life in adults with childhood-onset of Complex Regional Pain Syndrome type I.

Authors:	Tan EC; van de Sandt-Renkema N; Krabbe PF; Aronson DC; Severijnen RS
Institution:	Department of General Surgery-Traumatology, Radboud University Nijmegen Medical Centre, Nijmegen, The Netherlands. e.tan@chir.umcn.nl
Journal:	Injury. 2009 Aug;40(8):901-4. Epub 2009 Jun 13.
Abstract Link:	http://www.medifocus.com/abstracts.php?gid=NR015&ID=19524904

138.

Complex regional pain syndrome type 1 may be associated with menstrual cycle disorders: a case-control study.

Authors:	van den Berg I; Liem YS; Wesseldijk F; Zijlstra FJ; Hunink MG
Institution:	Department of Radiology, Erasmus University Medical Center Rotterdam, Rotterdam, The Netherlands. ineke.vandenberg@erasmusmc.nl
Journal:	Complement Ther Med. 2009 Oct-Dec;17(5-6):262-8. Epub 2009 Nov 7.
Abstract Link:	http://www.medifocus.com/abstracts.php?gid=NR015&ID=19942105

139.

Cortical reorganization in primary somatosensory cortex in patients with unilateral chronic pain.

Authors:	Vartiainen N; Kirveskari E; Kallio-Laine K; Kalso E; Forss N
Institution:	Brain Research Unit, Low Temperature Laboratory, Helsinki University of Technology, Espoo, Finland. nuutti@neuro.hut.fi
Journal:	J Pain. 2009 Aug;10(8):854-9.
Abstract Link:	http://www.medifocus.com/abstracts.php?gid=NR015&ID=19638329

Go to http://www.medifocus.com/links/NR015/0314 for direct online access to the above Abstract Links.

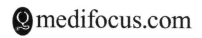

Drug Therapy Articles

140.

Treatment of Complex Regional Pain Syndrome (CRPS) using low dose naltrexone (LDN).

Authors:	Chopra P; Cooper MS
Institution:	Department of Medicine, Alpert Medical School of Brown University, 102 Smithfield Ave, Pawtucket, RI 02860, USA. painri@yahoo.com
Journal:	J Neuroimmune Pharmacol. 2013 Jun;8(3):470-6. doi: 10.1007/s11481-013-9451-y. Epub 2013 Apr 2.
Abstract Link:	http://www.medifocus.com/abstracts.php?gid=NR015&ID=23546884

141.

Predictors of pain relieving response to sympathetic blockade in complex regional pain syndrome type 1.

Authors:	van Eijs F; Geurts J; van Kleef M; Faber CG; Perez RS; Kessels AG; Van Zundert J
Institution:	Department of Anesthesiology and Pain Management, St. Elisabeth Hospital, Tilburg, The Netherlands. f.v.eys@elisabeth.nl
Journal:	Anesthesiology. 2012 Jan;116(1):113-21.
Abstract Link:	http://www.medifocus.com/abstracts.php?gid=NR015&ID=22143169

142.

Intramuscular botulinum toxin A (BtxA) in complex regional pain syndrome.

Authors:	Kharkar S; Ambady P; Yedatore V; Schwartzman RJ
Institution:	Hahnemann University Hospital, Philadelphia, PA , USA.
Journal:	Pain Physician. 2011 May-Jun;14(3):311-6.
Abstract Link:	http://www.medifocus.com/abstracts.php?gid=NR015&ID=21587336

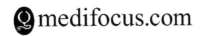

143.

Summaries for patients: Intravenous immunoglobulin treatment of the complex regional pain syndrome.

Author:
Journal: Ann Intern Med. 2010 Feb 2;152(3):I48.
Abstract Link: **ABSTRACT NOT AVAILABLE**

144.

Use of continuous interscalene brachial plexus block and rehabilitation to treat complex regional pain syndrome of the shoulder.

Authors: Detaille V; Busnel F; Ravary H; Jacquot A; Katz D; Allano G
Institution: CRRF Kerpape, 56275 Ploemeur cedex, France.
                 vdetaille@kerpape.mutualite56.fr
Journal: Ann Phys Rehabil Med. 2010 Aug-Sep;53(6-7):406-16. Epub 2010 Jul 2.
Abstract Link: http://www.medifocus.com/abstracts.php?gid=NR015&ID=20650698

145.

Opioid-sparing effect of intravenous outpatient ketamine infusions appears short-lived in chronic-pain patients with high opioid requirements.

Authors: Kapural L; Kapural M; Bensitel T; Sessler DI
Institution: Departments of Pain Management and Outcomes Research, Cleveland
                 Clinic, Cleveland, OH, USA. Kapural@ameritech.net
Journal: Pain Physician. 2010 Jul;13(4):389-94.
Abstract Link: http://www.medifocus.com/abstracts.php?gid=NR015&ID=20648208

Go to http://www.medifocus.com/links/NR015/0314 for direct online access to the above Abstract Links.

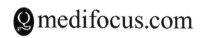
146.

The use of sub-anesthetic intravenous ketamine and adjuvant dexmedetomidine when treating acute pain from CRPS.

Authors:	Nama S; Meenan DR; Fritz WT
Institution:	Temple University School of Medicine, Philadelphia, PA, USA.
Journal:	Pain Physician. 2010 Jul;13(4):365-8.
Abstract Link:	http://www.medifocus.com/abstracts.php?gid=NR015&ID=20648205

147.

Botulinum toxin A (Botox) for treatment of proximal myofascial pain in complex regional pain syndrome: two cases.

Authors:	Safarpour D; Jabbari B
Institution:	Department of Neurology, Yale University School of Medicine, New Haven, Connecticut, USA. delaram.safarpour@yale.edu2
Journal:	Pain Med. 2010 Sep;11(9):1415-8. doi: 10.1111/j.1526-4637.2010.00929.x. Epub 2010 Aug 23.
Abstract Link:	http://www.medifocus.com/abstracts.php?gid=NR015&ID=20735753

148.

Intrathecal ziconotide for complex regional pain syndrome: seven case reports.

Authors:	Kapural L; Lokey K; Leong MS; Fiekowsky S; Stanton-Hicks M; Sapienza-Crawford AJ; Webster LR
Institution:	The Cleveland Clinic Foundation, Cleveland, Ohio 44195, USA. KAPURAL@ccf.org
Journal:	Pain Pract. 2009 Jul-Aug;9(4):296-303. Epub 2009 May 29.
Abstract Link:	http://www.medifocus.com/abstracts.php?gid=NR015&ID=19500276

Go to http://www.medifocus.com/links/NR015/0314 for direct online access to the above Abstract Links.

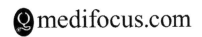

149.

Intrathecal glycine for pain and dystonia in complex regional pain syndrome.

Authors:	Munts AG; van der Plas AA; Voormolen JH; Marinus J; Teepe-Twiss IM; Onkenhout W; van Gerven JM; van Hilten JJ
Institution:	Department of Neurology, Leiden University Medical Center, P.O. Box 9600, 2300 RC Leiden, The Netherlands.
Journal:	Pain. 2009 Nov;146(1-2):199-204. Epub 2009 Aug 14.
Abstract Link:	http://www.medifocus.com/abstracts.php?gid=NR015&ID=19683392

150.

Efficacy of 5-day continuous lidocaine infusion for the treatment of refractory complex regional pain syndrome.

Authors:	Schwartzman RJ; Patel M; Grothusen JR; Alexander GM
Institution:	Department of Neurology, Drexel University College of Medicine, Philadelphia, Pennsylvania 19111-1839, USA. robert.schwartzman@drexelmed.edu
Journal:	Pain Med. 2009 Mar;10(2):401-12.
Abstract Link:	http://www.medifocus.com/abstracts.php?gid=NR015&ID=19284488

151.

Ketamine produces effective and long-term pain relief in patients with Complex Regional Pain Syndrome Type 1.

Authors:	Sigtermans MJ; van Hilten JJ; Bauer MC; Arbous MS; Marinus J; Sarton EY; Dahan A
Institution:	Department of Anesthesiology, Leiden University Medical Center, P.O. Box 9600, 2300 RC Leiden, The Netherlands.
Journal:	Pain. 2009 Oct;145(3):304-11. Epub 2009 Jul 14.
Abstract Link:	http://www.medifocus.com/abstracts.php?gid=NR015&ID=19604642

Go to http://www.medifocus.com/links/NR015/0314 for direct online access to the above Abstract Links.

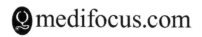

Clinical Trials Articles

152.

CT-guided stellate ganglion blockade vs. radiofrequency neurolysis in the management of refractory type I complex regional pain syndrome of the upper limb.

Authors:	Kastler A; Aubry S; Sailley N; Michalakis D; Siliman G; Gory G; Lajoie JL; Kastler B
Institution:	Radiology Department, University Hospital CHU Gabriel Montpied, 63000 Clermont-Ferrand, France. adriankastler@gmail.com
Journal:	Eur Radiol. 2013 May;23(5):1316-22. doi: 10.1007/s00330-012-2704-y. Epub 2012 Nov 9.
Abstract Link:	http://www.medifocus.com/abstracts.php?gid=NR015&ID=23138389

153.

Efficacy of intrathecal baclofen on different pain qualities in complex regional pain syndrome.

Authors:	van der Plas AA; van Rijn MA; Marinus J; Putter H; van Hilten JJ
Institution:	Department of Neurology, Leiden University Medical Center, PO Box 9600, 2300 RC Leiden, the Netherlands. A.A.van_der_Plas@lumc.nl
Journal:	Anesth Analg. 2013 Jan;116(1):211-5. doi: 10.1213/ANE.0b013e31826f0a2e. Epub 2012 Dec 7.
Abstract Link:	http://www.medifocus.com/abstracts.php?gid=NR015&ID=23223108

154.

Treatment of complex regional pain syndrome type I with neridronate: a randomized, double-blind, placebo-controlled study.

Authors:	Varenna M; Adami S; Rossini M; Gatti D; Idolazzi L; Zucchi F; Malavolta N; Sinigaglia L
Institution:	Rheumatology Unit, Ospedale G. Pini, Milan, Italy.
Journal:	Rheumatology (Oxford). 2013 Mar;52(3):534-42. doi: 10.1093/rheumatology/kes312. Epub 2012 Nov 30.
Abstract Link:	http://www.medifocus.com/abstracts.php?gid=NR015&ID=23204550

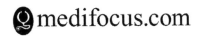

155.

Sensory signs in complex regional pain syndrome and peripheral nerve injury.

Authors: Gierthmuhlen J; Maier C; Baron R; Tolle T; Treede RD; Birbaumer N; Huge V; Koroschetz J; Krumova EK; Lauchart M; Maihofner C; Richter H; Westermann A

Institution: Division of Neurological Pain Research and Therapy, Department of Neurology, Universitatsklinikum Schleswig-Holstein, Campus Kiel, Kiel, Germany. j.gierthmuehlen@neurologie.uni-kiel.de

Journal: Pain. 2012 Apr;153(4):765-74. Epub 2011 Dec 10.

Abstract Link: http://www.medifocus.com/abstracts.php?gid=NR015&ID=22154921

156.

Using graded motor imagery for complex regional pain syndrome in clinical practice: failure to improve pain.

Authors: Johnson S; Hall J; Barnett S; Draper M; Derbyshire G; Haynes L; Rooney C; Cameron H; Moseley GL; de C Williams AC; McCabe C; Goebel A

Institution: The Walton Centre NHS Foundation Trust, Liverpool, L9 7LJ, UK.

Journal: Eur J Pain. 2012 Apr;16(4):550-61. doi: 10.1002/j.1532-2149.2011.00064.x. Epub 2011 Dec 19.

Abstract Link: http://www.medifocus.com/abstracts.php?gid=NR015&ID=22337591

157.

Therapeutic effect of acupuncture and massage for shoulder-hand syndrome in hemiplegia patients: a clinical two-center randomized controlled trial.

Authors: Li N; Tian F; Wang C; Yu P; Zhou X; Wen Q; Qiao X; Huang L

Institution: Acupuncture Department of Huaxi Hospital Affiliated to Sichuan University, Chengdu 610041, China.

Journal: J Tradit Chin Med. 2012 Sep;32(3):343-9.

Abstract Link: http://www.medifocus.com/abstracts.php?gid=NR015&ID=23297553

Go to http://www.medifocus.com/links/NR015/0314 for direct online access to the above Abstract Links.

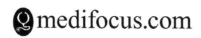

158.

Management of complex regional pain syndrome type I in upper extremity-evaluation of continuous stellate ganglion block and continuous infraclavicular brachial plexus block: a pilot study.

Authors: Toshniwal G; Sunder R; Thomas R; Dureja GP

Institution: Department of Anesthesiology, Wayne State University/Detroit Medical Center, Detroit, Michigan, USA. grtosh1@gmail.com

Journal: Pain Med. 2012 Jan;13(1):96-106. doi: 10.1111/j.1526-4637.2011.01285.x. Epub 2011 Dec 5.

Abstract Link: http://www.medifocus.com/abstracts.php?gid=NR015&ID=22142381

159.

The association between psychological factors and the development of complex regional pain syndrome type 1 (CRPS1)--a prospective multicenter study.

Authors: Beerthuizen A; Stronks DL; Huygen FJ; Passchier J; Klein J; Spijker AV

Institution: Department of Medical Psychology and Psychotherapy, Erasmus MC, Rotterdam, The Netherlands. a.beerthuizen@erasmusmc.nl

Journal: Eur J Pain. 2011 Oct;15(9):971-5. Epub 2011 Apr 2.

Abstract Link: http://www.medifocus.com/abstracts.php?gid=NR015&ID=21459637

160.

Work prognosis of complex regional pain syndrome type I: multicenter retrospective study on the determinants and time to return to work.

Authors: Dumas S; Pichon B; Dapolito AC; Bensefa-Colas L; Andujar P; Villa A; Descatha A

Journal: J Occup Environ Med. 2011 Dec;53(12):1354-6.

Abstract Link: **ABSTRACT NOT AVAILABLE**

Go to http://www.medifocus.com/links/NR015/0314 for direct online access to the above Abstract Links.

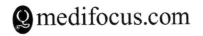
161.

Intravenous regional ketorolac and lidocaine in the treatment of complex regional pain syndrome of the lower extremity: a randomized, double-blinded, crossover study.

Authors:	Eckmann MS; Ramamurthy S; Griffin JG
Institution:	Department of Anesthesiology, University of Texas Health Science Center at San Antonio, San Antonio, TX 78229-3900, USA. eckmann@uthscsa.edu
Journal:	Clin J Pain. 2011 Mar-Apr;27(3):203-6.
Abstract Link:	http://www.medifocus.com/abstracts.php?gid=NR015&ID=21358290

162.

Drug-induced liver injury following a repeated course of ketamine treatment for chronic pain in CRPS type 1 patients: a report of 3 cases.

Authors:	Noppers IM; Niesters M; Aarts LP; Bauer MC; Drewes AM; Dahan A; Sarton EY
Institution:	Department of Anesthesiology, Leiden University Medical Center, Leiden, The Netherlands.
Journal:	Pain. 2011 Sep;152(9):2173-8. Epub 2011 May 4.
Abstract Link:	http://www.medifocus.com/abstracts.php?gid=NR015&ID=21546160

163.

The lack of efficacy of different infusion rates of intrathecal baclofen in complex regional pain syndrome: a randomized, double-blind, crossover study.

Authors:	van der Plas AA; Marinus J; Eldabe S; Buchser E; van Hilten JJ
Institution:	Department of Neurology, Leiden University Medical Center, Leiden, The Netherlands. A.A.van_der_Plas@lumc.nl
Journal:	Pain Med. 2011 Mar;12(3):459-65. doi: 10.1111/j.1526-4637.2011.01065.x. Epub 2011 Feb 18.
Abstract Link:	http://www.medifocus.com/abstracts.php?gid=NR015&ID=21332937

Go to http://www.medifocus.com/links/NR015/0314 for direct online access to the above Abstract Links.

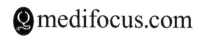

164.

Intravenous immunoglobulin treatment of the complex regional pain syndrome: a randomized trial.

Authors:	Goebel A; Baranowski A; Maurer K; Ghiai A; McCabe C; Ambler G
Institution:	University of Liverpool, Clinical Sciences Building, University Hospital Aintree, Liverpool L9 7AL, United Kingdom.
Journal:	Ann Intern Med. 2010 Feb 2;152(3):152-8.
Abstract Link:	http://www.medifocus.com/abstracts.php?gid=NR015&ID=20124231

165.

NMDA-receptor antagonist and morphine decrease CRPS-pain and cerebral pain representation.

Authors:	Gustin SM; Schwarz A; Birbaumer N; Sines N; Schmidt AC; Veit R; Larbig W; Flor H; Lotze M
Institution:	Institute of Medical Psychology and Behavioral Neurobiology, University of Tubingen, Germany.
Journal:	Pain. 2010 Oct;151(1):69-76. Epub 2010 Jul 13.
Abstract Link:	http://www.medifocus.com/abstracts.php?gid=NR015&ID=20630656

166.

Efficacy and safety of a single intrathecal methylprednisolone bolus in chronic complex regional pain syndrome.

Authors:	Munts AG; van der Plas AA; Ferrari MD; Teepe-Twiss IM; Marinus J; van Hilten JJ
Institution:	Department of Neurology, Leiden University Medical Center, P.O. Box 9600, 2300 RC Leiden, The Netherlands.
Journal:	Eur J Pain. 2010 May;14(5):523-8. Epub 2009 Dec 16.
Abstract Link:	http://www.medifocus.com/abstracts.php?gid=NR015&ID=20018535

Go to http://www.medifocus.com/links/NR015/0314 for direct online access to the above Abstract Links.

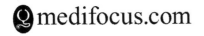

167.

Botulinum toxin A for treatment of allodynia of complex regional pain syndrome: a pilot study.

Authors:	Safarpour D; Salardini A; Richardson D; Jabbari B
Institution:	Department of Neurology, Yale University School of Medicine, New Haven, Connecticut, USA. delaram.safarpour@yale.edu
Journal:	Pain Med. 2010 Sep;11(9):1411-4. doi: 10.1111/j.1526-4637.2010.00897.x. Epub 2010 Jun 30.
Abstract Link:	http://www.medifocus.com/abstracts.php?gid=NR015&ID=20609130

168.

Brush-evoked allodynia predicts outcome of spinal cord stimulation in complex regional pain syndrome type 1.

Authors:	van Eijs F; Smits H; Geurts JW; Kessels AG; Kemler MA; van Kleef M; Joosten EA; Faber CG
Institution:	Maastricht University Medical Centre, Department of Anesthesiology and Pain Management, The Netherlands.
Journal:	Eur J Pain. 2010 Feb;14(2):164-9. Epub 2009 Nov 25.
Abstract Link:	http://www.medifocus.com/abstracts.php?gid=NR015&ID=19942463

169.

Effect of vitamin C on prevention of complex regional pain syndrome type I in foot and ankle surgery.

Authors:	Besse JL; Gadeyne S; Galand-Desme S; Lerat JL; Moyen B
Institution:	Universite de Lyon, Lyon, France. jean-luc.besse@chu-lyon.fr
Journal:	Foot Ankle Surg. 2009;15(4):179-82. Epub 2009 Apr 5.
Abstract Link:	http://www.medifocus.com/abstracts.php?gid=NR015&ID=19840748

Go to http://www.medifocus.com/links/NR015/0314 for direct online access to the above Abstract Links.

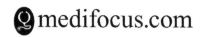

170.

Biphosphonates for the therapy of complex regional pain syndrome I--systematic review.

Authors: Brunner F; Schmid A; Kissling R; Held U; Bachmann LM
Institution: Department of Physical Medicine and Rheumatology, Balgrist University Hospital, Forchstrasse 340, 8008 Zurich, Switzerland. florian.brunner@balgrist.ch
Journal: Eur J Pain. 2009 Jan;13(1):17-21. Epub 2008 Apr 28.
Abstract Link: http://www.medifocus.com/abstracts.php?gid=NR015&ID=18440845

171.

Sympathetic block with botulinum toxin to treat complex regional pain syndrome.

Authors: Carroll I; Clark JD; Mackey S
Institution: Department of Anesthesiology, Stanford University School of Medicine, Stanford, CA 94304-1573, USA. irc39@pain.stanford.edu
Journal: Ann Neurol. 2009 Mar;65(3):348-51.
Abstract Link: http://www.medifocus.com/abstracts.php?gid=NR015&ID=19334078

172.

Intravenous magnesium for complex regional pain syndrome type 1 (CRPS 1) patients: a pilot study.

Authors: Collins S; Zuurmond WW; de Lange JJ; van Hilten BJ; Perez RS
Institution: Department of Anesthesiology, VU University Medical Center, Amsterdam, The Netherlands. s.collins@vumc.nl
Journal: Pain Med. 2009 Jul-Aug;10(5):930-40. Epub 2009 Jun 1.
Abstract Link: http://www.medifocus.com/abstracts.php?gid=NR015&ID=19496957

Go to http://www.medifocus.com/links/NR015/0314 for direct online access to the above Abstract Links.

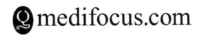

173.

Reduction of allodynia in patients with complex regional pain syndrome: A double-blind placebo-controlled trial of topical ketamine.

Authors: Finch PM; Knudsen L; Drummond PD
Institution: Perth Pain Management Centre, Perth, Australia; School of Psychology, Murdoch University, Perth, Australia.
Journal: Pain. 2009 Nov;146(1-2):18-25. Epub 2009 Aug 22.
Abstract Link: http://www.medifocus.com/abstracts.php?gid=NR015&ID=19703730

174.

Lumbar sympathetic blockade in children with complex regional pain syndromes: a double blind placebo-controlled crossover trial.

Authors: Meier PM; Zurakowski D; Berde CB; Sethna NF
Institution: Department of Anesthesiology, Perioperative and Pain Medicine, Children's Hospital Boston, Harvard Medical School, Boston, Massachusetts 02115, USA.
Journal: Anesthesiology. 2009 Aug;111(2):372-80.
Abstract Link: http://www.medifocus.com/abstracts.php?gid=NR015&ID=19602962

175.

Outpatient intravenous ketamine for the treatment of complex regional pain syndrome: a double-blind placebo controlled study.

Authors: Schwartzman RJ; Alexander GM; Grothusen JR; Paylor T; Reichenberger E; Perreault M
Institution: Department of Neurology, Drexel University College of Medicine, Philadelphia, PA 19102, USA. robert.schwartzman@drexelmed.edu
Journal: Pain. 2009 Dec 15;147(1-3):107-15. Epub 2009 Sep 23.
Abstract Link: http://www.medifocus.com/abstracts.php?gid=NR015&ID=19783371

Go to http://www.medifocus.com/links/NR015/0314 for direct online access to the above Abstract Links.

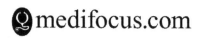

176.

Intrathecal baclofen for dystonia of complex regional pain syndrome.

Authors: van Rijn MA; Munts AG; Marinus J; Voormolen JH; de Boer KS;
                  Teepe-Twiss IM; van Dasselaar NT; Delhaas EM; van Hilten JJ

Institution: Department of Neurology, Leiden University Medical Center, P.O.
                  Box 9600, 2300 RC Leiden, The Netherlands.

Journal: Pain. 2009 May;143(1-2):41-7. Epub 2009 Feb 18.

Abstract Link: http://www.medifocus.com/abstracts.php?gid=NR015&ID=19232828

177.

Complex regional pain syndrome type I: efficacy of stellate ganglion blockade.

Authors: Yucel I; Demiraran Y; Ozturan K; Degirmenci E

Institution: Department of Orthopaedics and Traumatology, University of Duzce,
                  Duzce, Turkey. istemiyucel@yahoo.com

Journal: J Orthop Traumatol. 2009 Dec;10(4):179-83. Epub 2009 Nov 4.

Abstract Link: http://www.medifocus.com/abstracts.php?gid=NR015&ID=19888550

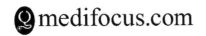

Nerve Block Articles

178.

Sympathetic nerve blocks, pragmatic trials, and responder analysis.

Authors:	Sethna NF; Berde CB
Journal:	Anesthesiology. 2012 Jan;116(1):12-4.
Abstract Link:	**ABSTRACT NOT AVAILABLE**

179.

Interventional management of intractable sympathetically mediated pain by computed tomography-guided catheter implantation for block and neuroablation of the thoracic sympathetic chain: technical approach and review of 322 procedures.

Authors:	Agarwal-Kozlowski K; Lorke DE; Habermann CR; Schulte am Esch J; Beck H
Institution:	Centre for Palliative Care and Pain Management (T.I.P.S!), Stade, Germany.
Journal:	Anaesthesia. 2011 Aug;66(8):699-708. doi: 10.1111/j.1365-2044.2011.06765.x. Epub 2011 May 13.
Abstract Link:	http://www.medifocus.com/abstracts.php?gid=NR015&ID=21564048

180.

Stellate ganglion blockade (SGB) for refractory index finger pain - a case report.

Authors:	Hey M; Wilson I; Johnson MI
Institution:	Pain Management Services, Mid Yorkshire Hospitals NHS Trust, The Boothroyd Day Centre, Dewsbury & District Hospital, Dewsbury, WF13 4HS, West Yorkshire, United Kingdom. martin.hey@midyorks.nhs.uk
Journal:	Ann Phys Rehabil Med. 2011 May;54(3):181-8. Epub 2011 Apr 13.
Abstract Link:	http://www.medifocus.com/abstracts.php?gid=NR015&ID=21493175

Go to http://www.medifocus.com/links/NR015/0314 for direct online access to the above Abstract Links.

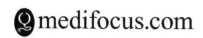

181.

Complex regional pain syndrome type I as a consequence of trauma or surgery to upper extremity: management with intravenous regional anaesthesia, using lidocaine and methyloprednisolone.

Authors: Varitimidis SE; Papatheodorou LK; Dailiana ZH; Poultsides L; Malizos KN

Institution: Department of Orthopaedic Surgery, University of Thessalia School of Medicine, Larissa, Greece. svaritimidis@ortho-uth.org

Journal: J Hand Surg Eur Vol. 2011 Nov;36(9):771-7. Epub 2011 Jun 30.

Abstract Link: http://www.medifocus.com/abstracts.php?gid=NR015&ID=21719518

182.

Use of regional blockade to facilitate inpatient rehabilitation of recalcitrant complex regional pain syndrome.

Authors: Carayannopoulos AG; Cravero JP; Stinson MT; Sites BD

Institution: Department of Neurosurgery, Lahey Clinic, Burlington, MA 02142, USA. Alexios.G.Carayannopoulos@lahey.org

Journal: PM R. 2009 Feb;1(2):194-8.

Abstract Link: **ABSTRACT NOT AVAILABLE**

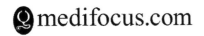

Electrical Stimulation Articles

183.

Spinal cord stimulation in complex regional pain syndrome type I of less than 12-month duration.

Authors:	van Eijs F; Geurts JW; Van Zundert J; Faber CG; Kessels AG; Joosten EA; van Kleef M
Institution:	Department of Anesthesiology and Pain Therapy, St Elisabeth Hospital, Tilburg, The Netherlands.
Journal:	Neuromodulation. 2012 Mar-Apr;15(2):144-50; discussion 150. doi: 10.1111/j.1525-1403.2011.00424.x. Epub 2012 Feb 13.
Abstract Link:	http://www.medifocus.com/abstracts.php?gid=NR015&ID=22329446

184.

Pain relief and functional recovery in patients with complex regional pain syndrome after motor cortex stimulation.

Authors:	Fonoff ET; Hamani C; Ciampi de Andrade D; Yeng LT; Marcolin MA; Jacobsen Teixeira M
Institution:	Department of Neurology, Division of Functional Neurosurgery of the Institute of Psychiatry, University of Sao Paulo School of Medicine, Sao Paulo, Brazil. fonoffet@usp.br
Journal:	Stereotact Funct Neurosurg. 2011;89(3):167-72. Epub 2011 Apr 13.
Abstract Link:	http://www.medifocus.com/abstracts.php?gid=NR015&ID=21494069

185.

Spinal cord stimulation is effective in management of complex regional pain syndrome I: fact or fiction.

Authors:	Kumar K; Rizvi S; Bnurs SB
Institution:	Section of Neurosurgery, Department of Surgery, Regina General Hospital, University of Saskatchewan, Regina, Saskatchewan, Canada. krishna.kumar@rqhealth.ca
Journal:	Neurosurgery. 2011 Sep;69(3):566-78; discussion 5578-80.
Abstract Link:	http://www.medifocus.com/abstracts.php?gid=NR015&ID=21441839

Go to http://www.medifocus.com/links/NR015/0314 for direct online access to the above Abstract Links.

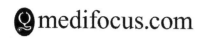

186.

Motor cortex stimulation for trigeminal neuropathic or deafferentation pain: an institutional case series experience.

Authors: Raslan AM; Nasseri M; Bahgat D; Abdu E; Burchiel KJ
Institution: Department of Neurological Surgery, Oregon Health & Science University, Portland, OR 97239, USA.
Journal: Stereotact Funct Neurosurg. 2011 Apr;89(2):83-8. Epub 2011 Feb 2.
Abstract Link: http://www.medifocus.com/abstracts.php?gid=NR015&ID=21293167

187.

Overview of complex regional pain syndrome and recent management using spinal cord stimulation.

Author: Hyatt KA
Institution: kayhyatt@gmail.com
Journal: AANA J. 2010 Jun;78(3):208-12.
Abstract Link: http://www.medifocus.com/abstracts.php?gid=NR015&ID=20572407

188.

Peripheral neuromodulation for pain.

Authors: Bittar RG; Teddy PJ
Institution: Department of Neurosurgery, Royal Melbourne Hospital, Parkville, Victoria, Australia. drbittar@precisionneurosurgery.com
Journal: J Clin Neurosci. 2009 Oct;16(10):1259-61. Epub 2009 Jun 28.
Abstract Link: http://www.medifocus.com/abstracts.php?gid=NR015&ID=19564116

Go to http://www.medifocus.com/links/NR015/0314 for direct online access to the above Abstract Links.

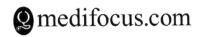

189.

Can the outcome of spinal cord stimulation in chronic complex regional pain syndrome type I patients be predicted by catastrophizing thoughts?

Authors: Lame IE; Peters ML; Patijn J; Kessels AG; Geurts J; van Kleef M
Institution: Department of Pain Management, ResearchCentre, University Hospital
                  Maastricht, The Netherlands. ingelame@telfort.n
Journal: Anesth Analg. 2009 Aug;109(2):592-9.
Abstract Link: http://www.medifocus.com/abstracts.php?gid=NR015&ID=19608836

190.

Effect of spinal cord stimulation in Type I complex regional pain syndrome with 2 rare severe cutaneous manifestations.

Authors: Rijkers K; van Aalst J; Kurt E; Daemen MA; Beuls EA; Spincemaille
                  GH
Institution: Department of Neurosurgery, Maastricht University Hospital,
                  Maastricht, The Netherlands. kimrijkers@gmail.com
Journal: J Neurosurg. 2009 Feb;110(2):274-8.
Abstract Link: http://www.medifocus.com/abstracts.php?gid=NR015&ID=18928361

191.

Motor cortex electrical stimulation applied to patients with complex regional pain syndrome.

Authors: Velasco F; Carrillo-Ruiz JD; Castro G; Arguelles C; Velasco AL;
                  Kassian A; Guevara U
Institution: Unit for Stereotactic, Functional Neurosurgery and Radiosurgery of the
                  Service of Neurology and Neurosurgery and Pain Clinic, General
                  Hospital of Mexico, Mexico City, Mexico.
Journal: Pain. 2009 Sep 28.
Abstract Link: http://www.medifocus.com/abstracts.php?gid=NR015&ID=19793621

Go to http://www.medifocus.com/links/NR015/0314 for direct online access to the above Abstract Links.

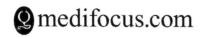

Spinal cord stimulation: "neural switch" in complex regional pain syndrome type I.

Authors:	Williams KA; Korto K; Cohen SP
Institution:	Department of Anesthesiology and Critical Care Medicine, Johns Hopkins School of Medicine, 550North Broadway Suite 309A, Baltimore, MD 21205, USA. kwilli64@jhmi.edu
Journal:	Pain Med. 2009 May-Jun;10(4):762-6.
Abstract Link:	http://www.medifocus.com/abstracts.php?gid=NR015&ID=19638145

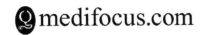

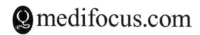

NOTES

Use this page for taking notes as you review your Guidebook

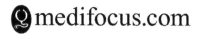

4 - Centers of Research

This section of your *MediFocus Guidebook* is a unique directory of doctors, researchers, medical centers, and research institutions with specialized research interest, and in many cases, clinical expertise in the management of this specific medical condition. The *Centers of Research* directory is a valuable resource for quickly identifying and locating leading medical authorities and medical institutions within the United States and other countries that are considered to be at the forefront in clinical research and treatment of this disorder.

Use the *Centers of Research* directory to contact, consult, or network with leading experts in the field and to locate a hospital or medical center that can help you.

The following information is provided in the *Centers of Research* directory:

- **Geographic Location**

    - United States: the information is divided by individual states listed in alphabetical order. Not all states may be included.

    - Other Countries: information is presented for select countries worldwide listed in alphabetical order. Not all countries may be included.

- **Names of Authors**

    - Select names of individual authors (doctors, researchers, or other health-care professionals) with specialized research interest, and in many cases, clinical expertise in the management of this specific medical condition, who have recently published articles in leading medical journals about the condition.

    - E-mail addresses for individual authors, if listed on their specific publications, is also provided.

- **Institutional Affiliations**

    - Next to each individual author's name is their **institutional affiliation** (hospital, medical center, or research institution) where the study was conducted as listed in their publication(s).

- In many cases, information about the specific **department** within the medical institution where the individual author was located at the time the study was conducted is also provided.

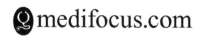
Centers of Research

United States

AL - Alabama

Name of Author	Institutional Affiliation
Kirchner JS	Division of Orthopaedic Surgery, University of Alabama at Birmingham, Birmingham, AL 35205-5327, USA. dr.shah.ashish@gmail.com
Shah A	Division of Orthopaedic Surgery, University of Alabama at Birmingham, Birmingham, AL 35205-5327, USA. dr.shah.ashish@gmail.com

AZ - Arizona

Name of Author	Institutional Affiliation
Kautz DD	Midwestern University, Glendale, AZ, USA.
Montana C	Midwestern University, Glendale, AZ, USA.

CA - California

Name of Author	Institutional Affiliation
Altmaier EM	Psychology Service, VA Palo Alto Health Care System, (116B), 3801 Miranda Ave., Palo Alto, CA, USA, jessica-lohnberg@uiowa.edu
Altschuler EL	Center for Brain and Cognition, University of California, San Diego, 9500 Gilman Drive, 0109, La Jolla, California 92093-0109, USA. vramacha@ucsd.edu
Carroll I	Department of Anesthesiology, Stanford University School of Medicine, Stanford, CA 94304-1573, USA. irc39@pain.stanford.edu
Clark JD	Department of Anesthesia, Stanford University, Palo Alto, California, USA.

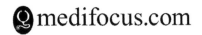

Hsu ES	Pain Management Center, Department of Anesthesiology, David Geffen School of Medicine, University of California, Los Angeles, LA, USA. ehsu@mednet.ucla.edu
Ilfeld BM	Clinical Investigation, University of California San Diego, 200 West Arbor Dr., MC 8770, San Diego, CA 92103-8770, USA. bilfeld@ucsd.edu
Lohnberg JA	Psychology Service, VA Palo Alto Health Care System, (116B), 3801 Miranda Ave., Palo Alto, CA, USA, jessica-lohnberg@uiowa.edu
Mackey S	Department of Anesthesiology, Stanford University School of Medicine, Stanford, CA 94304-1573, USA. irc39@pain.stanford.edu
Pepper A	Department of Anesthesia, Stanford University, Palo Alto, California, USA.
Prager JP	Center for the Rehabilitation of Pain Syndromes (CRPS), UCLA Medical Plaza, Department of Anesthesiology, David Geffen School of Medicine at UCLA, Los Angeles, California 90095, USA. joshuaprager@gmail.com
Ramachandran VS	Center for Brain and Cognition, University of California, San Diego, 9500 Gilman Drive, 0109, La Jolla, California 92093-0109, USA. vramacha@ucsd.edu

CT - Connecticut

Name of Author	Institutional Affiliation
Jabbari B	Department of Neurology, Yale University School of Medicine, New Haven, Connecticut, USA. delaram.safarpour@yale.edu2
Safarpour D	Department of Neurology, Yale University School of Medicine, New Haven, Connecticut, USA. delaram.safarpour@yale.edu2

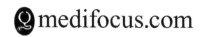

DC - Washington D.C.

Name of Author	Institutional Affiliation
Kogan M	Physician Assistant Program, George Washington Center for Integrative Medicine, Washington, DC, USA.
Lamont K	Physician Assistant Program, George Washington Center for Integrative Medicine, Washington, DC, USA.

FL - Florida

Name of Author	Institutional Affiliation
Crick BC	North Florida Surgeons, St. Vincent's Medical Center, 1 Shircliff Way St., Jacksonville, Florida, 32204, USA.
Crick JC	North Florida Surgeons, St. Vincent's Medical Center, 1 Shircliff Way St., Jacksonville, Florida, 32204, USA.

IL - Illinois

Name of Author	Institutional Affiliation
Bruehl S	Center for Pain Studies, Rehabilitation Institute of Chicago, Illinois 60611, USA. nharden@ric.org
Carlson RM	Section of Podiatry, Department of Orthopedic Surgery, Loyola University Medical Center, Maywood, IL, USA.
Harden RN	Rehabilitation Institute of Chicago, Department of Physical Medicine and Rehabilitation, Northwestern University Feinberg School of Medicine, Chicago, Illinois, USA. chris.ramsden@nih.gov
Harris EJ	Section of Podiatry, Department of Orthopedic Surgery, Loyola University Medical Center, Maywood, IL, USA.
Ramsden C	Rehabilitation Institute of Chicago, Department of Physical Medicine and Rehabilitation, Northwestern University Feinberg School of Medicine, Chicago, Illinois, USA. chris.ramsden@nih.gov
Vatine JJ	Rehabilitation Institute of Chicago, Chicago, IL 60611, USA. nharden@ric.org

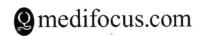
IN - Indiana

Name of Author	Institutional Affiliation
Compton AK	SMC Pain Center, Schneck Medical Center, 411 West Tipton Street, Seymour, IN 47274, USA.
Hayek SM	SMC Pain Center, Schneck Medical Center, 411 West Tipton Street, Seymour, IN 47274, USA.

KY - Kentucky

Name of Author	Institutional Affiliation
Cappello ZJ	School of Medicine and Division of Plastic Surgery, University of Louisville, Louisville, KY, USA. zjcapp01@louisville.edu
Louis DS	School of Medicine and Division of Plastic Surgery, University of Louisville, Louisville, KY, USA. zjcapp01@louisville.edu

MA - Massachussetts

Name of Author	Institutional Affiliation
Aner M	Pain Medicine at Harvard Medical School, Beth Israel Deaconess Medical Center, Boston, Massachusetts 07503, USA. bmjakubowicz@gmail.com
Berde CB	Division of Pain Medicine, Department of Anesthesiology, Periperative and Pain Medicine, Children's Hospital, Boston, Massachusetts 02115, USA. deridre.logan@childrens.harvard.edu
Borsook D	P.A.I.N. group, Department of Psychiatry, McLean Hospital, Belmont, MA, USA.
Carayannopoulos AG	Department of Neurosurgery, Lahey Clinic, Burlington, MA 02142, USA. Alexios.G.Carayannopoulos@lahey.org
Fields HL	Department of Neurology, Massachusetts General Hospital, Harvard Medical School, Boston, MA 02114, USA. aoaklander@partners.org

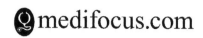
Jakubowicz B	Pain Medicine at Harvard Medical School, Beth Israel Deaconess Medical Center, Boston, Massachusetts 07503, USA. bmjakubowicz@gmail.com
Logan DE	Division of Pain Medicine, Department of Anesthesiology, Periperative and Pain Medicine, Children's Hospital, Boston, Massachusetts 02115, USA. deridre.logan@childrens.harvard.edu
Meier PM	Department of Anesthesiology, Perioperative and Pain Medicine, Children's Hospital Boston, Harvard Medical School, Boston, Massachusetts 02115, USA.
Oaklander AL	Department of Neurology, Massachusetts General Hospital, Harvard Medical School, Boston, MA 02114, USA. aoaklander@partners.org
Sava S	P.A.I.N. group, Department of Psychiatry, McLean Hospital, Belmont, MA, USA.
Sethna NF	Department of Anesthesiology, Perioperative and Pain Medicine, Children's Hospital Boston, Harvard Medical School, Boston, Massachusetts 02115, USA.
Sites BD	Department of Neurosurgery, Lahey Clinic, Burlington, MA 02142, USA. Alexios.G.Carayannopoulos@lahey.org
Wurtman RJ	Massachusetts Institute of Technology, Cambridge, MA 02139, USA. dick@mit.edu

MD - Maryland

Name of Author	Institutional Affiliation
Cohen SP	Department of Anesthesiology and Critical Care Medicine, Johns Hopkins School of Medicine, 550North Broadway Suite 309A, Baltimore, MD 21205, USA. kwilli64@jhmi.edu
Dellon L	Johns Hopkins University, Baltimore, MD, USA. ALDellon@Dellon.com
Krasna MJ	Program of Health Policy, St. Joseph Cancer Institute, University of Maryland, 7501 Osler Drive, Suite 104, Towson, MD 21204, USA. markkrasna@catholichealth.net

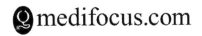

Raja SN	Division of Pain Medicine, Department of Anesthesiology and Critical Care Medicine at Johns Hopkins University School of Medicine, Baltimore, MD 21287, USA.
Rosson GD	Johns Hopkins University, Baltimore, MD, USA. ALDellon@Dellon.com
Williams KA	Department of Anesthesiology and Critical Care Medicine, Johns Hopkins School of Medicine, 550North Broadway Suite 309A, Baltimore, MD 21205, USA. kwilli64@jhmi.edu

MI - Michigan

Name of Author	Institutional Affiliation
Dureja GP	Department of Anesthesiology, Wayne State University/Detroit Medical Center, Detroit, Michigan, USA. grtosh1@gmail.com
Toshniwal G	Department of Anesthesiology, Wayne State University/Detroit Medical Center, Detroit, Michigan, USA. grtosh1@gmail.com

MO - Missouri

Name of Author	Institutional Affiliation
Cruz N	Department of Psychology, St. Louis Children's Hospital, One Children's Place, St. Louis, MO 63118, USA. nxc2032@bjc.org
Ruamwijitphong W	DePaul Health Center, Bridgeton, MO, USA.
Salorio CF	Department of Psychology, St. Louis Children's Hospital, One Children's Place, St. Louis, MO 63118, USA. nxc2032@bjc.org

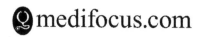

NC - North Carolina

Name of Author	Institutional Affiliation
Andrew Koman L	Department of Orthopaedic Surgery, Wake Forest University School of Medicine, Wake Forest University Health Sciences, Medical Center Boulevard, Winston-Salem, NC 27157, USA.
Azari P	Department of Anesthesiology, Division of Pain Management, Duke University School of Medicine, Durham, NC 27710, USA.
Chang JC	Coastal Carolina Neuropsychiatric Center, Jacksonville, NC, USA.
Edwards CL	Departments of Psychiatry double daggerHematology daggerDuke Pain and Palliative Care Clinic, Duke University Medical Center, Durham, NC 27705, USA. feliu001@mc.duke.edu
Feliu MH	Departments of Psychiatry double daggerHematology daggerDuke Pain and Palliative Care Clinic, Duke University Medical Center, Durham, NC 27705, USA. feliu001@mc.duke.edu
Koman LA	Department of Orthopaedic Surgery, Wake Forest University School of Medicine, Winston-Salem, NC 27157, USA.
Leversedge FJ	Department of Orthopaedic Surgery, Duke University, DUMC Box 2836, Durham, NC 27710, USA. fraser.leversedge@duke.edu
Li Z	Department of Orthopaedic Surgery, Wake Forest University School of Medicine, Wake Forest University Health Sciences, Medical Center Boulevard, Winston-Salem, NC 27157, USA.
Patterson RW	Department of Orthopaedic Surgery, Wake Forest University School of Medicine, Winston-Salem, NC 27157, USA.
Pyati S	Department of Anesthesiology, Division of Pain Management, Duke University School of Medicine, Durham, NC 27710, USA.

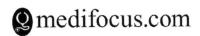

| Sprague M | Coastal Carolina Neuropsychiatric Center, Jacksonville, NC, USA. |
| Srinivasan RC | Department of Orthopaedic Surgery, Duke University, DUMC Box 2836, Durham, NC 27710, USA. fraser.leversedge@duke.edu |

NY - New York

Name of Author	Institutional Affiliation
Epstein LJ	Department of Anesthesiology, Mount Sinai School of Medicine, New York, NY, USA. lawrence.epstein@mountsinai.org
Palmieri M	Department of Anesthesiology, Mount Sinai School of Medicine, New York, NY, USA. lawrence.epstein@mountsinai.org
Raja SN	Department of Anesthesiology, College of Physicians & Surgeons of Columbia University, New York, NY, USA.
Sharma A	Department of Anesthesiology, College of Physicians & Surgeons of Columbia University, New York, NY, USA.

OH - Ohio

Name of Author	Institutional Affiliation
Chae J	Department of Physical Medicine and Rehabilitation, Case Western Reserve University, Cleveland, Ohio, USA.
Goldschneider KR	Cincinnati Children's Hospital Medical Center, Cincinnati, OH, USA. kenneth.goldschneider@cchmc.org
Janata JW	Departments of Psychiatry and Anesthesiology, University Hospitals Case Medical Center, Cleveland, OH 44106, USA.
Kapural L	The Cleveland Clinic Foundation, Cleveland, Ohio 44195, USA. KAPURAL@ccf.org
Martin DP	Department of aAnesthesiology and Pain Medicine, Nationwide Children's Hospital and the Ohio State University, Columbus, Ohio 43205, USA.

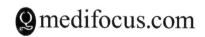

Sessler DI	Departments of Pain Management and Outcomes Research, Cleveland Clinic, Cleveland, OH, USA. Kapural@ameritech.net
Stanton-Hicks M	Pain Management Department, Center for Neurological Restoration, Consulting Staff, Children's Hospital CCF Shaker Campus, Pediatric Pain Rehabilitation Program, Cleveland Clinic, Cleveland, Ohio 44195, USA. stantom@ccf.org
Tobias JD	Department of aAnesthesiology and Pain Medicine, Nationwide Children's Hospital and the Ohio State University, Columbus, Ohio 43205, USA.
Veizi IE	Departments of Psychiatry and Anesthesiology, University Hospitals Case Medical Center, Cleveland, OH 44106, USA.
Webster LR	The Cleveland Clinic Foundation, Cleveland, Ohio 44195, USA. KAPURAL@ccf.org

OR - Oregon

Name of Author	Institutional Affiliation
Burchiel KJ	Department of Neurological Surgery, Oregon Health & Science University, Portland, OR 97239, USA.
Ochoa JL	The Oregon Nerve Center, Good Samaritan Medical Center, 1040 NW 22nd Ave., Suite 600, Portland, OR 97210, USA. jochoa@nervesense.net
Raslan AM	Department of Neurological Surgery, Oregon Health & Science University, Portland, OR 97239, USA.
Verdugo RJ	The Oregon Nerve Center, Good Samaritan Medical Center, 1040 NW 22nd Ave., Suite 600, Portland, OR 97210, USA. jochoa@nervesense.net

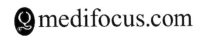

PA - Pennsylvania

Name of Author	Institutional Affiliation
Alexander GM	Department of Neurology, Drexel University College of Medicine, Philadelphia, Pennsylvania 19111-1839, USA. robert.schwartzman@drexelmed.edu
Falowski S	St. Lukes Neurosurgical Associates, St. Lukes University Hospital, Bethlehem, PA, USA.
Fritz WT	Temple University School of Medicine, Philadelphia, PA, USA.
Grothusen JR	Department of Neurology, Drexel University College of Medicine, PA, USA. robert.schwartzman@drexelmed.edu
Kalanuria A	Department of Neurology, Drexel University, College of Medicine, Philadelphia, PA 19102, USA. dlibon@Drexelmed.edu
Kanter AS	Department of Neurological Surgery, University of Pittsburgh Medical Center, Pittsburgh, Pennsylvania.
Kharkar S	Hahnemann University Hospital, Philadelphia, PA and Department of Neurology, Drexel University College of Medicine, Philadelphia, PA 19107, USA.
Libon DJ	Department of Neurology, Drexel University, College of Medicine, Philadelphia, PA 19102, USA. dlibon@Drexelmed.edu
Morr S	Department of Neurological Surgery, University of Pittsburgh Medical Center, Pittsburgh, Pennsylvania.
Nama S	Temple University School of Medicine, Philadelphia, PA, USA.
Perreault M	Department of Neurology, Drexel University College of Medicine, Philadelphia, PA 19102, USA. robert.schwartzman@drexelmed.edu
Peterlin BL	Department of Neurology, Drexel University College of Medicine, Philadelphia, PA, USA.
Schwartzman RJ	Department of Cardiology, Drexel University College of Medicine, Philadelphia, Pennsylvania, USA. doctorjay21074@yahoo.com

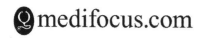

Sharan A	St. Lukes Neurosurgical Associates, St. Lukes University Hospital, Bethlehem, PA, USA.
Smith JA	Department of Cardiology, Drexel University College of Medicine, Philadelphia, Pennsylvania, USA. doctorjay21074@yahoo.com

RI - Rhode Island

Name of Author	Institutional Affiliation
Chopra P	Department of Medicine, Alpert Medical School of Brown University, 102 Smithfield Ave, Pawtucket, RI 02860, USA. painri@yahoo.com
Cooper MS	Department of Medicine, Alpert Medical School of Brown University, 102 Smithfield Ave, Pawtucket, RI 02860, USA. painri@yahoo.com

TN - Tennessee

Name of Author	Institutional Affiliation
Bruehl S	Department of Anesthesiology, Vanderbilt University School of Medicine, Nashville, Tennessee 37212, USA. stephen.bruehl@vanderbilt.edu

TX - Texas

Name of Author	Institutional Affiliation
Eckmann MS	Department of Anesthesiology, University of Texas Health Science Center at San Antonio, San Antonio, TX 78229-3900, USA. eckmann@uthscsa.edu
Edmondson EA	Department of Neurology, Baylor College of Medicine, Houston, Texas, USA.
Griffin JG	Department of Anesthesiology, University of Texas Health Science Center at San Antonio, San Antonio, TX 78229-3900, USA. eckmann@uthscsa.edu
Hommer DH	Physical Medicine and Rehabilitation Service, Department of Orthopedics and Rehabilitation, Brooke Army Medical Center, 3551 Roger Brooke Drive, Fort Sam Houston, TX

78234, USA.

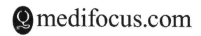

Jupiter DC	Texas A&M Health and Science Center, College of Medicine, Temple, TX, USA. shibuya@medicine.tamhsc.edu
Shibuya N	Texas A&M Health and Science Center, College of Medicine, Temple, TX, USA. shibuya@medicine.tamhsc.edu
Shirani P	Department of Neurology, Baylor College of Medicine, Houston, Texas, USA.

VA - Virginia

Name of Author	Institutional Affiliation
Gonzales M	Division of Endocrinology and Metabolism, Department of Internal Medicine, Strelitz Center for Diabetes and Endocrine Disorders, Eastern Virginia Medical School, 855 West Brambleton Avenue, Norfolk, VA 23510, USA.
Khardori R	Division of Endocrinology and Metabolism, Department of Internal Medicine, Strelitz Center for Diabetes and Endocrine Disorders, Eastern Virginia Medical School, 855 West Brambleton Avenue, Norfolk, VA 23510, USA.

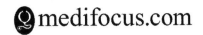

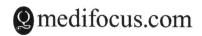

Centers of Research

Other Countries

Australia

Name of Author	Institutional Affiliation
Bialocerkowski AE	Department of Physiotherapy, Austin Hospital, Heidelberg 3084, Victoria, Australia. anne.daly@austin.org.au
Bittar RG	Department of Neurosurgery, Royal Melbourne Hospital, Parkville, Victoria, Australia. drbittar@precisionneurosurgery.com
Daly A	School of Biomedical and Health Sciences, University of Western Sydney, Sydney, Australia. a.bialocerkowski@uws.edu.au
Daly AE	Department of Physiotherapy, Austin Hospital, Heidelberg 3084, Victoria, Australia. anne.daly@austin.org.au
Drummond PD	Perth Pain Management Centre, Perth, Australia; School of Psychology, Murdoch University, Perth, Australia.
Finch PM	Perth Pain Management Centre, Perth, Australia; School of Psychology, Murdoch University, Perth, Australia.
Miao EY	M. Modern TCM Clinic , Melbourne, Victoria, Australia .
Moseley GL	Neuroscience Research Australia, University of New South Wales, Sydney, Australia.
O'Connell NE	Neuroscience Research Australia, Randwick, Australia.
Parkitny L	Neuroscience Research Australia, University of New South Wales, Sydney, Australia.
Stanton TR	Neuroscience Research Australia, Randwick, Australia.
Teddy PJ	Department of Neurosurgery, Royal Melbourne Hospital, Parkville, Victoria, Australia. drbittar@precisionneurosurgery.com

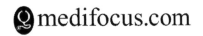

Brazil

Name of Author	Institutional Affiliation
Fonoff ET	Department of Neurology, Division of Functional Neurosurgery of the Institute of Psychiatry, University of Sao Paulo School of Medicine, Sao Paulo, Brazil. fonoffet@usp.br
Jacobsen Teixeira M	Department of Neurology, Division of Functional Neurosurgery of the Institute of Psychiatry, University of Sao Paulo School of Medicine, Sao Paulo, Brazil. fonoffet@usp.br

Canada

Name of Author	Institutional Affiliation
Blaise GA	Multinnova Medical Centre, Universite de Montreal, Montreal, QC, Canada.
Blake DR	McGill University, Montreal, Canada. jenslewis@hotmail.com
Bnurs SB	Section of Neurosurgery, Department of Surgery, Regina General Hospital, University of Saskatchewan, Regina, Saskatchewan, Canada. krishna.kumar@rqhealth.ca
Coderre TJ	Department of Anesthesia and Alan Edward Centre for Research on Pain, McGill University, and McGill University Health Centre Research Institute, Montreal, Quebec.
Finlayson RJ	Department of Anesthesia, Montreal General Hospital, McGill University, Montreal, H3G 1A4, Quebec, Canada. de_tran@hotmail.com
Kumar K	Section of Neurosurgery, Department of Surgery, Regina General Hospital, University of Saskatchewan, Regina, Saskatchewan, Canada. krishna.kumar@rqhealth.ca
Lagueux E	Faculty of Medicine and Health Sciences, University of Sherbrooke, Quebec, Canada.
Lewis JS	McGill University, Montreal, Canada. jenslewis@hotmail.com

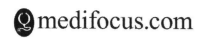

Schweinhardt P	Faculty of Dentistry, McGill University, Montreal, Canada. jenslewis@hotmail.com
Taha R	Multinnova Medical Centre, Universite de Montreal, Montreal, QC, Canada.
Tousignant-Laflamme Y	Faculty of Medicine and Health Sciences, University of Sherbrooke, Quebec, Canada.
Tran de QH	Department of Anesthesia, Montreal General Hospital, McGill University, Montreal, H3G 1A4, Quebec, Canada. de_tran@hotmail.com

China

Name of Author	**Institutional Affiliation**
Huang L	Acupuncture Department of Huaxi Hospital Affiliated to Sichuan University, Chengdu 610041, China.
Li N	Acupuncture Department of Huaxi Hospital Affiliated to Sichuan University, Chengdu 610041, China.

Finland

Name of Author	**Institutional Affiliation**
Forss N	Brain Research Unit, Low Temperature Laboratory, Helsinki University of Technology, Espoo, Finland. nuutti@neuro.hut.fi
Vartiainen N	Brain Research Unit, Low Temperature Laboratory, Helsinki University of Technology, Espoo, Finland. nuutti@neuro.hut.fi

France

Name of Author	**Institutional Affiliation**
Allano G	CRRF Kerpape, 56275 Ploemeur cedex, France. vdetaille@kerpape.mutualite56.fr
Besse JL	Universite de Lyon, Lyon, France. jean-luc.besse@chu-lyon.fr

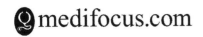

Detaille V	CRRF Kerpape, 56275 Ploemeur cedex, France. vdetaille@kerpape.mutualite56.fr
Kastler A	Radiology Department, University Hospital CHU Gabriel Montpied, 63000 Clermont-Ferrand, France. adriankastler@gmail.com
Kastler B	Radiology Department, University Hospital CHU Gabriel Montpied, 63000 Clermont-Ferrand, France. adriankastler@gmail.com
Moyen B	Universite de Lyon, Lyon, France. jean-luc.besse@chu-lyon.fr

Germany

Name of Author	Institutional Affiliation
Agarwal-Kozlowski K	Centre for Palliative Care and Pain Management (T.I.P.S!), Stade, Germany.
Azad SC	Department of Anaesthesiology, Ludwig-Maximilians-Universitat Munchen, Munich, Germany. vhuge@med.uni-muenchen.de
Baron R	Division of Neurological Pain Research and Therapy, Department of Neurology, University Hospital Schleswig-Holstein, Campus Kiel, Arnold-Heller-Str. 3, Haus 41, 24105, Kiel, Germany. d.naleschinski@neurologie.uni-kiel.de
Beck H	Centre for Palliative Care and Pain Management (T.I.P.S!), Stade, Germany.
Bernateck M	Department of Anesthesiology, Pain Clinic, Hannover Medical School, Carl-Neuberg-Str. 1, Hannover 30625, Germany. bernateck.michael@mh-hannover.de
Birklein F	Department of Neurology, Johannes Gutenberg University, Langenbeckstrasse 1, 55101 Mainz, Germany. eberlet@uni-mainz.de
Brunkhorst T	Department of Anesthesiology, Pain Clinic, Hannover Medical School, Carl-Neuberg-Str. 1, Hannover 30625, Germany. bernateck.michael@mh-hannover.de

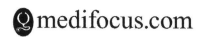

Eberle T	Department of Neurology, Johannes Gutenberg University, Langenbeckstrasse 1, 55101 Mainz, Germany. eberlet@uni-mainz.de
Gierthmuhlen J	Division of Neurological Pain Research and Therapy, Department of Neurology, Universitatsklinikum Schleswig-Holstein, Campus Kiel, Kiel, Germany. j.gierthmuehlen@neurologie.uni-kiel.de
Gustin SM	Institute of Medical Psychology and Behavioral Neurobiology, University of Tubingen, Germany.
Huge V	Department of Anaesthesiology, Ludwig-Maximilians-Universitat Munchen, Munich, Germany. vhuge@med.uni-muenchen.de
Janig W	Physiologisches Institut, Christian-Albrechts-Universitat zu Kiel, Kiel, Germany. w.janig@physiologie.uni-kiel.de
Knoeller SM	Department of Orthopaedic and Trauma Surgery, University Hospital Freiburg, Freiburg, Germany. stefan.knoeller@uniklinik-freiburg.de
Kolb L	Department of Neurology, University Hospital Erlangen, Erlangen, Germany.
Lotze M	Institute of Medical Psychology and Behavioral Neurobiology, University of Tubingen, Germany.
Maihofner C	Department of Neurology, University Hospital Erlangen, Erlangen, Germany.
McQuay HJ	Department of Occupational and Social Medicine, University of Gottingen, Waldweg 37 B, Gottingen, Germany, D-37073.
Naleschinski D	Division of Neurological Pain Research and Therapy, Department of Neurology, University Hospital Schleswig-Holstein, Campus Kiel, Arnold-Heller-Str. 3, Haus 41, 24105, Kiel, Germany. d.naleschinski@neurologie.uni-kiel.de
Schurmann M	Department of Orthopedic Surgery, University of Bochum, Germany. t.vogel@klinikum-bochum.de
Straube S	Department of Occupational and Social Medicine, University of Gottingen, Waldweg 37 B, Gottingen, Germany, D-37073.

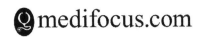

Vogel T	Department of Orthopedic Surgery, University of Bochum, Germany. t.vogel@klinikum-bochum.de
Wasner G	Department of Neurology, Division of Neurological Pain Research and Therapy, University Clinic of Schleswig-Holstein, Kiel, Germany. g.wasner@neurologie.uni-kiel.de
Westermann A	Division of Neurological Pain Research and Therapy, Department of Neurology, Universitatsklinikum Schleswig-Holstein, Campus Kiel, Kiel, Germany. j.gierthmuehlen@neurologie.uni-kiel.de
Wolter T	Department of Orthopaedic and Trauma Surgery, University Hospital Freiburg, Freiburg, Germany. stefan.knoeller@uniklinik-freiburg.de

Greece

Name of Author	**Institutional Affiliation**
Malizos KN	Department of Orthopaedic Surgery, University of Thessalia School of Medicine, Larissa, Greece. svaritimidis@ortho-uth.org
Varitimidis SE	Department of Orthopaedic Surgery, University of Thessalia School of Medicine, Larissa, Greece. svaritimidis@ortho-uth.org

Italy

Name of Author	**Institutional Affiliation**
Cabitza P	Dipartimento Di Scienze Medico-Chirurgiche, Universita Degli Studi Di Milano, IRCCS Policlinico San Donato, Milan, Italy.
Cacchio A	Department of Physical Medicine and Rehabilitation, "San Salvatore" Hospital of L'Aquila, L'Aquila, Italy,angelo.cacchio@tin.it.
Fiore P	Department of Physical Medicine and Rehabilitation, University of Foggia, Foggia, Italy.

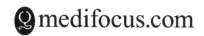

Randelli P	Dipartimento Di Scienze Medico-Chirurgiche, Universita Degli Studi Di Milano, IRCCS Policlinico San Donato, Milan, Italy.
Santamato A	Department of Physical Medicine and Rehabilitation, University of Foggia, Foggia, Italy.
Sinigaglia L	Rheumatology Unit, Ospedale G. Pini, Milan, Italy.
Spacca G	Department of Physical Medicine and Rehabilitation, "San Salvatore" Hospital of L'Aquila, L'Aquila, Italy,angelo.cacchio@tin.it.
Varenna M	Rheumatology Unit, Ospedale G. Pini, Milan, Italy.

Japan

Name of Author	Institutional Affiliation
Morita K	Department of Anesthesiology and Resuscitology, Okayama University Graduate School of Medicine and Dentistry, Okayama City, Okayama Prefecture, 700-8551, Japan. tento@cc.okayama-u.ac.jp
Sato K	Department of Anesthesiology and Resuscitology, Okayama University Graduate School of Medicine and Dentistry, Okayama City, Okayama Prefecture, 700-8551, Japan. tento@cc.okayama-u.ac.jp

Korea

Name of Author	Institutional Affiliation
Ahn RS	Department of Anesthesiology and Pain Medicine, The Armed Forces Capital Hospital, Seoul, Republic of Korea.
Park JY	Department of Anesthesiology and Pain Medicine, The Armed Forces Capital Hospital, Seoul, Republic of Korea.

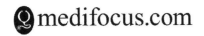

Mexico

Name of Author	Institutional Affiliation
Guevara U	Unit for Stereotactic, Functional Neurosurgery and Radiosurgery of the Service of Neurology and Neurosurgery and Pain Clinic, General Hospital of Mexico, Mexico City, Mexico.
Velasco F	Unit for Stereotactic, Functional Neurosurgery and Radiosurgery of the Service of Neurology and Neurosurgery and Pain Clinic, General Hospital of Mexico, Mexico City, Mexico.

Netherlands

Name of Author	Institutional Affiliation
Beek PJ	Research Institute MOVE, Faculty of Human Movement Sciences, VU University Amsterdam, van der Boechorststraat 9, 1081 BT Amsterdam, The Netherlands.
Beerthuizen A	Department of Medical Psychology and Psychotherapy, Erasmus MC, Rotterdam, The Netherlands. a.beerthuizen@erasmusmc.nl
Bodde MI	Department of Rehabilitation Medicine, University Medical Center Groningen, P.O. Box 30.001, 9700 RB Groningen, The Netherlands. m.i.bodde@rev.umcg.nl
Collins S	Department of Anesthesiology, VU University Medical Center, Amsterdam, The Netherlands. s.collins@vumc.nl
Dahan A	Department of Anesthesiology, Leiden University Medical Center, P.O. Box 9600, 2300 RC Leiden, The Netherlands.
Dirckx M	Erasmus MC, Rotterdam, The Netherlands. m.dirckx@erasmusmc.nl
Ek JW	Department of Rehabilitation Medicine, Bethesda Hospital, Hoogeveen.
Ezendam D	Center for Human Movement Sciences, University of Groningen, University Medical Center Groningen, Groningen, The Netherlands.

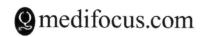

Faber CG	Maastricht University Medical Centre, Department of Anesthesiology and Pain Management, The Netherlands.
Fischer SG	Department of Anesthesiology, VU University Medical Center, Amsterdam, The Netherlands. s.fischer@vumc.nl
Frolke JP	Department of Rehabilitation, Nijmegen Centre of Evidence Based Practice, Radboud University Nijmegen Medical Centre, Nijmegen, The Netherlands. h.vandemeent@reval.umcn.nl
Geertzen JH	VU University Medical Center, Department of Anaesthesiology, Amsterdam, the Netherlands. rsgm.perez@vumc.nl
Goris RJ	Department of Surgery, Radboud University Nijmegen Medical Centre, Nijmegen, The Netherlands. E.Tan@chir.umcn.nl
Groeneweg G	Department of Anesthesiology, Subdivision Pain Treatment Centre, Erasmus MC, Rotterdam, The Netherlands. j.groeneweg@erasmusmc.nl
Hulsman NM	Centre for Rehabilitation, University Medical Centre Groningen, University of Groningen, PO Box 30001, 9700 RB Groningen, The Netherlands. n.m.hulsman@rev.umcg.nl
Hunink MG	Department of Radiology, Erasmus University Medical Center Rotterdam, Rotterdam, The Netherlands. ineke.vandenberg@erasmusmc.nl
Huygen F	Department of Anesthesiology and Pain Therapy, St. Elisabeth Hospital, Tilburg, The Netherlands.
Huygen FJ	Erasmus University Medical Center, Pharmaco-epidemiology Unit, Departments of Medical Informatics and Epidemiology & Biostatistics, Rotterdam, The Netherlands. m.vrolijk-demos@erasmusmc.nl
Jannink MJ	Center for Human Movement Sciences, University of Groningen, University Medical Center Groningen, Groningen, The Netherlands.
Lame IE	Department of Pain Management, ResearchCentre, University Hospital Maastricht, The Netherlands. ingelame@telfort.n

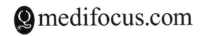

Marinus J	Department of Neurology, Leiden University Medical Center, Leiden, The Netherlands.
Munts AG	Department of Neurology, Leiden University Medical Center, P.O. Box 9600, 2300 RC, Leiden, The Netherlands.
Noppers IM	Department of Anesthesiology, Leiden University Medical Center, Leiden, The Netherlands.
Patijn J	Department of Rehabilitation, University Hospital Maastricht, Maastricht, The Netherlands. jeroen.dejong@mumc.nl
Perez RS	Department of Anesthesiology, VU University Medical Center, Amsterdam, The Netherlands. rdh.deboer@vumc.nl
Rijkers K	Department of Neurosurgery, Maastricht University Hospital, Maastricht, The Netherlands. kimrijkers@gmail.com
Rothgangel AS	The Department of Health and Technique, Zuyd University of Applied Sciences, Heerlen, The Netherlands. a.s.rothgangel@hszuyd.nl
Sarton EY	Department of Anesthesiology, Leiden University Medical Center, Leiden, The Netherlands.
Severijnen RS	Department of General Surgery-Traumatology, Radboud University Nijmegen Medical Centre, Nijmegen, The Netherlands. e.tan@chir.umcn.nl
Sigtermans MJ	Department of Anesthesiology, Leiden University Medical Center, P.O. Box 9600, 2300 RC Leiden, The Netherlands.
Spijker AV	Department of Medical Psychology and Psychotherapy, Erasmus MC, Rotterdam, The Netherlands. a.beerthuizen@erasmusmc.nl
Spincemaille GH	Department of Neurosurgery, Maastricht University Hospital, Maastricht, The Netherlands. kimrijkers@gmail.com
Sturkenboom MC	Pharmaco-Epidemiology Unit, Department of Medical Informatics and Epidemiology & Biostatistics, Erasmus University Medical Center, Rotterdam, The Netherlands. m.vrolijk-demos@erasmusmc.nl

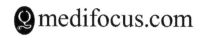

Swart CM	Research Institute MOVE, Faculty of Human Movement Sciences, VU University Amsterdam, van der Boechorststraat 9, 1081 BT Amsterdam, The Netherlands.
Tan EC	Department of Surgery, Radboud University Nijmegen Medical Centre, Nijmegen, The Netherlands. E.Tan@chir.umcn.nl
Van Bodegraven Hof EA	Department of Anesthesiology, Pain Treatment Centre, Erasmus MC, Rotterdam, the Netherlands.
Van Zundert J	Department of Anesthesiology and Pain Management, St. Elisabeth Hospital, Tilburg, The Netherlands. f.v.eys@elisabeth.nl
Wade DT	The Department of Health and Technique, Zuyd University of Applied Sciences, Heerlen, The Netherlands. a.s.rothgangel@hszuyd.nl
Zijlstra FJ	Department of Anesthesiology, Pain Treatment Centre, Erasmus MC, Rotterdam, the Netherlands.
de Boer RD	Department of Anesthesiology, VU University Medical Center, Amsterdam, The Netherlands. rdh.deboer@vumc.nl
de Jong JR	Department of Rehabilitation, University Hospital Maastricht, Maastricht, The Netherlands. jeroen.dejong@mumc.nl
de Mos M	Pharmaco-Epidemiology Unit, Department of Medical Informatics and Epidemiology & Biostatistics, Erasmus University Medical Center, Rotterdam, The Netherlands. m.vrolijk-demos@erasmusmc.nl
de Rooij AM	Department of Neurology, Leiden University Medical Center, Leiden, The Netherlands.
den Dunnen WF	Centre for Rehabilitation, University Medical Centre Groningen, University of Groningen, PO Box 30001, 9700 RB Groningen, The Netherlands. n.m.hulsman@rev.umcg.nl
van Dongen RT	Department of Rehabilitation Medicine, Bethesda Hospital, Hoogeveen.
van Eijs F	Maastricht University Medical Centre, Department of Anesthesiology and Pain Management, The Netherlands.

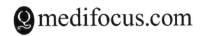

van Hilten JJ	Department of Neurology, Leiden University Medical Center, PO Box 9600, 2300 RC Leiden, the Netherlands. A.A.van_der_Plas@lumc.nl
van Kleef M	Department of Anesthesiology and Pain Therapy, St Elisabeth Hospital, Tilburg, The Netherlands.
van Rijn MA	Department of Neurology, Leiden University Medical Center, P.O. Box 9600, 2300 RC Leiden, The Netherlands.
van de Meent H	Department of Rehabilitation, Nijmegen Centre of Evidence Based Practice, Radboud University Nijmegen Medical Centre, Nijmegen, The Netherlands. h.vandemeent@reval.umcn.nl
van den Berg I	Department of Radiology, Erasmus University Medical Center Rotterdam, Rotterdam, The Netherlands. ineke.vandenberg@erasmusmc.nl
van der Plas AA	Department of Neurology, Leiden University Medical Center, PO Box 9600, 2300 RC Leiden, the Netherlands. A.A.van_der_Plas@lumc.nl

Poland

Name of Author	**Institutional Affiliation**
Puchalski P	Department of General and Hand Surgery, Pomeranian Medical University in Szczecin, Szczecin, Poland. azyluk@hotmail.com
Zyluk A	Department of General and Hand Surgery, Pomeranian Medical University in Szczecin, Szczecin, Poland. azyluk@hotmail.com

Switerland

Name of Author	**Institutional Affiliation**
Luthi F	Clinique Romande de Readaptation SuvaCare, avenue Grand-Champsec 90, 1951 Sion, Switzerland. aurelie.vouilloz@crr-suva.ch
Vouilloz A	Clinique Romande de Readaptation SuvaCare, avenue Grand-Champsec 90, 1951 Sion, Switzerland. aurelie.vouilloz@crr-suva.ch

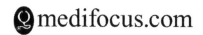 **medifocus.com**

Switzerland

Name of Author	Institutional Affiliation
Bachmann LM	Department of Physical Medicine and Rheumatology, Balgrist University Hospital, Forchstrasse 340, CH-8008 Zurich, Switzerland. florian.brunner@balgrist.ch
Brunner F	Horten Center for Patient Oriented Research and Knowledge Transfer, Department of Internal Medicine, University of Zurich, Pestalozzistrasse 24, CH-8032 Zurich, Switzerland.
Konzelmann M	Department for musculoskeletal rehabilitation, Clinique romande de readaptation suvacare, 90 avenue du grand champsec, Sion 1951, Switzerland. Michel.konzelmann@crr-suva.ch
Luthi F	Department for musculoskeletal rehabilitation, Clinique romande de readaptation suvacare, 90 avenue du grand champsec, Sion 1951, Switzerland. Michel.konzelmann@crr-suva.ch
Wertli M	Horten Center for Patient Oriented Research and Knowledge Transfer, Department of Internal Medicine, University of Zurich, Pestalozzistrasse 24, CH-8032 Zurich, Switzerland.

Turkey

Name of Author	Institutional Affiliation
Akalin E	Department of Physical Medicine and Rehabilitation, Dokuz Eylul University Faculty of Medicine, Inciralti, Izmir, Turkey. banudilek1979@gmail.com
Alpayci M	Yuzuncu Yil University Medical Faculty, Physical Medicine and Rehabilitation Department, 65100 Van, Turkey. leventediz@gmail.com
Cerci SS	Department of Physical Medicine and Rehabilitation, Suleyman Demirel University Medical School, Isparta, Turkey. serpilsavas@yahoo.com

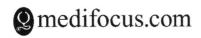

Degirmenci E	Department of Orthopaedics and Traumatology, University of Duzce, Duzce, Turkey. istemiyucel@yahoo.com
Dilek B	Department of Physical Medicine and Rehabilitation, Dokuz Eylul University Faculty of Medicine, Inciralti, Izmir, Turkey. banudilek1979@gmail.com
Dincer K	Department of Physical Medicine and Rehabilitation, Gulhane Military Medical Academy, Etlik, 06018, Ankara, Turkey. iltekinduman@yahoo.com
Duman I	Department of Physical Medicine and Rehabilitation, Gulhane Military Medical Academy, Etlik, 06018, Ankara, Turkey. iltekinduman@yahoo.com
Ediz L	Yuzuncu Yil University Medical Faculty, Physical Medicine and Rehabilitation Department, 65100 Van, Turkey. leventediz@gmail.com
Savas S	Department of Physical Medicine and Rehabilitation, Suleyman Demirel University Medical School, Isparta, Turkey. serpilsavas@yahoo.com
Yucel I	Department of Orthopaedics and Traumatology, University of Duzce, Duzce, Turkey. istemiyucel@yahoo.com

United Kingdom

Name of Author	Institutional Affiliation
Agrawal SK	Department of Paediatric Neurology, Sheffield Children's Hospital, Sheffield, UK.
Ambler G	University of Liverpool, Clinical Sciences Building, University Hospital Aintree, Liverpool L9 7AL, United Kingdom.
Bailey J	Bath Centre for Pain Services, The Royal National Hospital for Rheumatic Diseases, Upper Borough Walls, Bath BA1 1RL, UK.
Blake D	Department of Psychology, University of Bath, UK. psskr@bath.ac.uk
Butchart AG	Department of Anaesthesia, Norfolk & Norwich University Hospital, Norwich, Norfolk, UK. angusbutchart@doctors.org.uk

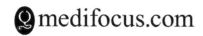

Cossins L	Pain Research Institute, Clinical Sciences Centre, University Hospital Aintree, Liverpool, UK.
Field J	Cheltenham General Hospital, Cheltenham, UK. jeremy.field@glos.nhs.uk
Goebel A	King's College London School of Medicine.
Hey M	Pain Management Services, Mid Yorkshire Hospitals NHS Trust, The Boothroyd Day Centre, Dewsbury & District Hospital, Dewsbury, WF13 4HS, West Yorkshire, United Kingdom. martin.hey@midyorks.nhs.uk
Johnson MI	Pain Management Services, Mid Yorkshire Hospitals NHS Trust, The Boothroyd Day Centre, Dewsbury & District Hospital, Dewsbury, WF13 4HS, West Yorkshire, United Kingdom. martin.hey@midyorks.nhs.uk
Johnson S	The Walton Centre NHS Foundation Trust, Liverpool, L9 7LJ, UK.
Kunnumpurath S	St George's School of Anaesthesia, Tooting, London, UK. dreeku@doctors.org.uk
Lee J	Pain Management Centre, National Hospital for Neurology & Neurosurgery, Queen Square, London.
McCabe CS	Bath Centre for Pain Services, The Royal National Hospital for Rheumatic Diseases, Upper Borough Walls, Bath BA1 1RL, UK.
Mordekar SR	Department of Paediatric Neurology, Sheffield Children's Hospital, Sheffield, UK.
Moseley GL	Department of Physiology, Anatomy & Genetics, University of Oxford, Oxford, UK. lorimer.moseley@gmail.com
Nandi P	Pain Management Centre, National Hospital for Neurology & Neurosurgery, Queen Square, London.
Regan L	Department of Psychology, University of Bath, Bath, UK. psskr@bath.ac.uk
Rodham K	Department of Psychology, University of Bath, UK. psskr@bath.ac.uk
Surendran A	Department of Anaesthesia, Norfolk & Norwich University Hospital, Norwich, Norfolk, UK. angusbutchart@doctors.org.uk

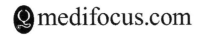

Turner-Stokes L   King's College London School of Medicine.

Vadivelu N   St George's School of Anaesthesia, Tooting, London, UK. dreeku@doctors.org.uk

Wiech K   Department of Physiology, Anatomy & Genetics, University of Oxford, Oxford, UK. lorimer.moseley@gmail.com

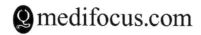

NOTES

Use this page for taking notes as you review your Guidebook

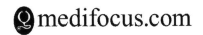

5 - Tips on Finding and Choosing a Doctor

Introduction

One of the most important decisions confronting patients who have been diagnosed with a serious medical condition is finding and choosing a qualified physician who will deliver a high level and quality of medical care in accordance with currently accepted guidelines and standards of care. Finding the "best" doctor to manage your condition, however, can be a frustrating and time-consuming experience unless you know what you are looking for and how to go about finding it.

The process of finding and choosing a physician to manage your specific illness or condition is, in some respects, analogous to the process of making a decision about whether or not to invest in a particular stock or mutual fund. After all, you wouldn't invest your hard eared money in a stock or mutual fund without first doing exhaustive research about the stock or fund's past performance, current financial status, and projected future earnings. More than likely you would spend a considerable amount of time and energy doing your own research and consulting with your stock broker before making an informed decision about investing. The same general principle applies to the process of finding and choosing a physician. Although the process requires a considerable investment in terms of both time and energy, the potential payoff can be well worth it--after all, what can be more important than your health and well-being?

This section of your Guidebook offers important tips for how to find physicians as well as suggestions for how to make informed choices about choosing a doctor who is right for you.

Tips for Finding Physicians

Finding a highly qualified, competent, and compassionate physician to manage your specific illness or condition takes a lot of hard work and energy but is an investment that is well-worth the effort. It is important to keep in mind that you are not looking for just any general physician but rather for a physician who has expertise in the treatment and management of your specific illness or condition. Here are some suggestions for where you can turn to identify and locate physicians who specialize in managing your disorder:

- **Your Doctor** - Your family physician (family medicine or internal medicine specialist) is a good starting point for finding a physician who specializes in your illness. Chances are that your doctor already knows several specialists in your geographic area who specialize in your illness and can recommend several names to you. Your doctor can also provide you with information about their qualifications, training, and hospital affiliations.

- **Your Peer Network** - Your family, friends, and co-workers can be a potentially very useful network for helping you find a physician who specializes in your illness. They may know someone else with this condition and may be able to put you in touch with them to find out which doctors they can recommend. If you have friends, neighbors, or relatives who work in hospitals (e.g., nurses, social workers, administrators), they may be a potentially valuable source for helping you find a physician who specializes in your condition.

- **Hospitals and Medical Centers** - Hospitals and medical centers are, potentially, an excellent source for finding physicians who specialize in treating specific diseases. Simply contact hospitals and major medical centers in your city, county, or state and ask if they have anyone on their staff who specializes in treating your condition. When you call, ask to speak to someone in the specific Department that cares for patients with the illness. For example, if you have been diagnosed with cancer, ask to speak with someone in the Department of Hematology and Oncology. If you are not sure which Department treats patients with your specific condition, ask to speak to someone in the Department of Medicine since this Department is the umbrella for many other medical specialties.

- **Organizations and Support Groups** - Many disease organizations and support groups that cater to patients with a specific illness or condition maintain physician referral lists and may be able to recommend doctors in your geographic area who specialize in the treatment and management of your specific disorder. This *MediFocus Guidebook* includes a select listing of disease organizations and support groups that you may wish to contact to ask for a physician referral.

- **Managed Care Plans** - If you belong to a managed care plan, you can obtain a list of physicians who belong to the Plan from the plan's membership services office. Keep in mind, however, that your choices will usually be limited to only those doctors who belong to the Plan. If you decide to go outside the Plan, you will likely have to pay for the doctor's services "out of pocket".

- **Medical Journals** - Many doctors based at major medical centers and universities who have special interest in a particular disease or condition conduct research and publish their findings in leading medical journals. Searching the medical literature can help you identify and locate leading physicians who are recognized as experts in their field about a particular illness. This *MediFocus Guidebook* includes an extensive listing of the names and institutional affiliations of physicians and researchers, in the United States and other countries, who have recently published their studies about this specific medical condition in leading medical journals. You can also conduct your own online search for your illness or condition and identify additional authors and hospitals who specialize in the disease using the PubMed database available at http://www.nlm.nih.gov.

- **American Medical Association** - The American Medical Association (AMA) is the nation's largest professional medical association that represents many doctors in the United States and also provides a free physician locator service called "AMA Physician Select" available at http://dbapps.ama-assn.org/aps/amahg.htm. You can search the AMA database by either "Physician Name" or "Medical Specialty". You can find information about physicians including medical school and residency training, area of specialty, and contact information.

- **American Board of Medical Specialists** - The American Board of Medical Specialists (ABMS) publishes a geographical list of board-certified physicians called the Official ABMS Directory of Board Certified Medical Specialists that is available in most public libraries. Physicians who are listed in the ABMS Directory are board-certified in a medical specialty meaning that they have passed rigorous certification examinations administered by a board of medical specialists. There are 24 specialty boards that are recognized by the ABMS and the AMA. Each candidate applying for board certification must pass a written examination given by the specific specialty board and 15 of the specialty boards also require candidates to pass an oral examination in order to obtain board certification. To find out if a particular physician you are considering is board certified:

  - Visit your local public library and ask for a copy of the Official ABMS Directory of Board Certified Medical Specialists.

  - Search the ABMS web site at http://www.abms.org/login.asp.

  - Call the ABMS toll free at 1-866-275-2267.

- **American Society of Clinical Oncology** - The American Society of Clinical Onclology (ASC)) is the largest professional organization that represents physicians who specialize in treating cancer patients (oncologists). The ASCO provides a searchable database of ASCO members called "Find an Oncologist" that you can access online at http://www.asco.org. You can search the "Find an Oncologist" database for a cancer specialist by name, city, state, country, or specialty area.

- **American Cancer Society** - The American Cancer Society (ACS) is a nationwide voluntary health organization dedicated to helping cancer patients and survivors through research, education, advocacy, and services. The ACS web site http://www.cancer.org is not only an excellent resource for cancer information but also includes a "Message Board" where you can ask questions, exchange ideas, and share stories. The ACS Message Board is also a potentially useful source for locating an oncologist in your geographical area who specializes in your specific type of cancer. You can also contact the ACS toll free by calling 1-800-ACS-2345.

- **National Comprehensive Cancer Network** - The National Comprehensive Cancer Network (NCCN) is an alliance of 19 of the world's leading cancer centers and is dedicated to helping patients and health care professionals make informed decisions about cancer care. You can find a listing of the 19 NCCN member cancer institutions on the NCCN web site at http://www.nccn.org/. You can also search the NCCN "Physician Directory" for doctors located at any of the 19 NCCN member cancer institutions at http://www.nccn.org/physician_directory/SearchPers.asp. This database is an excellent resource for locating leading cancer specialists nationwide who specialize in your specific type of cancer.

- **National Cancer Institute Clinical Trials Database** - The National Cancer Institute (NCI) is part of the National Institutes of Health (NIH) and coordinates the National Cancer Program which conducts and supports research, training, and a variety of other programs dedicated to prevention and treatment of cancer. The NCI maintains an extensive cancer clinical trials database that you can access at http://www.cancer.gov/clinicaltrials. You can search the database for current clinical trials by type of cancer and even limit your search to clinical trials within you geographical area by putting in your Zip Code. The NCI clinical trials database also provides contact information for the physicians who serve as the study coordinators for each clinical trial. This database is a valuable resource for identifying and locating leading physicians in your local area and around the country who are conducting cutting-edge clinical research about your specific type of cancer.

- **National Center for Complementary and Alternative Medicine** - The National Center for Complementary and Alternative Medicine (NCCAM) is part of the National Institutes of Health (NIH) and is dedicated to exploring complementary and alternative medicine healing practices in the context of rigorous scientific research and methodology. The NCCAM web site http://nccam.nih.gov/ includes publications, frequently asked questions, and useful links to other complementary and alternative medicine resources. If you have questions about complementary and alternative medicine practices for your particular illness or medical condition, you can contact

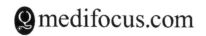

the NCCAM Clearinghouse toll-free in the U.S. at 1-888-644-6226 or 301-519-3153. You can also contact the NCCAM Clearinghouse by E-mail: info@nccam.nih.gov.

- **National Organization for Rare Disorders** - The National Organization for Rare Disorders (NORD) is a federation of voluntary health organizations dedicated to helping patients with rare "orphan" diseases and their families. There are over 6,000 rare or "orphan" diseases that are estimated to affect approximately 25 million Americans. You can search NORD's "Rare Diseases Database" for information about rare diseases at http://www.rarediseases.org/search/rdblist.html. In addition to providing useful information about rare diseases, NORD maintains a confidential "Networking Program" for its members to enable them to communicate with other patients who suffer from the same disorder. To learn more about NORD's Networking Program, you can send an E mail to: orphan@rarediseases.org.

How to Make Informed Choices About Physicians

It has generally been assumed by many people that the longer a physician has been in practice, the more experience, knowledge, and skills he/she has accumulated and, therefore, the higher the quality of care they provide to their patients. Recent research conducted by a group of doctors from the Harvard Medical School, however, seems to strongly suggest that this premise may not be true. In an article published in February 2005 in the *Annals of Internal Medicine* (Volume 142, No. 4, pp. 260-303), the Harvard researchers seriously challenged the common assumption that the more clinical experience a physician has accumulated, the higher the level of medical care they provide to their patients.

In fact, surprisingly, the researchers found an inverse (opposite) relationship between the number of years that a physician has been in practice (i.e., experience) and the quality of care that the physician provides. In other words, the widely held belief that "practice makes perfect" does not necessarily apply to all physicians and should not be the sole criteria used by patients in their decision analysis for choosing a physician. The underlying message of this study is that the length of time a physician has been in practice does not necessarily equate to a high quality of medical care unless the doctor takes steps to keep abreast with new advances and changing patterns of clinical practice.

Here are some important issues you need to consider and carefully research before making an informed decision about choosing your doctor:

- **Board Certification** - Board certified doctors are required to have extra training after medical school to become specialists in a particular field of medicine and are required to take continuing education courses in order to maintain their board certification status. Check with the American Board of Medical Specialists (ABMS) to determine if a specific physician you are considering is board certified in a particular medical specialty. To find out if a particular physician you are considering is board certified:

  - Visit your local public library and ask for a copy of the Official ABMS Directory of Board Certified Medical Specialists.

  - Search the ABMS web site at http://www.abms.org/login.asp.

  - Call the ABMS toll free at 1-866-275-2267.

- **Experience** - As noted above, research from the Harvard Medical School strongly suggests that how long a physician has been in practice (i.e., experience) does not necessarily correlate with a high level of medical care. The most important issue, therefore, is not how long a doctor has been in practice but rather how much experience the physician has in treating your specific illness or medical condition. Some physicians who have been in practice for many decades may have only treated a small number of patients with the specific disorder, whereas, some younger physicians who have been in practice only a few years may have already treated hundreds of patients with the same disorder. Here are some suggestions for helping you find out about a particular physician's experience in treating your specific illness:

  - Call the physician's office and speak with a staff member such as a nurse or physician's assistant. Ask them for information about how many patients with your specific medical condition the physician treats during the course of a year. Ask how many patients with this condition the physician is currently treating. You will have to call several different physicians' offices in order to have a basis for comparing the numbers of patients.

  - Find out if the physician has published any articles about the condition in reputable medical journals by doing an author search online. You can conduct an online author search using PubMed at http://www.nlm.nih.gov. Simply click on the "PubMed" icon, select the "author" field from the "Limits" menu, enter the physician's name (last name followed by first initial), and then click on the "Go" button. The author search will retrieve all articles published by the particular physician you are considering.

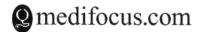

- Talk with your family physician and ask if he/she can provide you with any information about the particular physician's experience in treating patients with your specific illness or condition.

- Contact disease organizations and support groups that specialize in helping patients with your specific disorder and ask if they can provide you with any information, including experience, about the physician you are considering.

- **Medical School Affiliation** - Find out if the physician you are considering also has a joint faculty appointment at a medical school. In general, practicing community physicians with a joint academic appointment at a medical school are more likely to be in contact with leading medical experts and may be more up-to-date with the latest advances in research and treatments than community based physicians who are not affiliated with a medical school.

- **Hospital Affiliation** - Find out about the hospitals that the doctor uses. In the event that you need to be treated at a hospital, is the hospital where the physician has admitting privileges nearby to your home or will you (and your family members) have to travel a considerable distance?

- **Hospital Accreditation** - Find out if the hospital where the physician has admitting privileges is accredited by the Joint Commission on Accreditation of Healthcare Organizations (JCAHO). You can find information about a specific hospital's accreditation status by searching the JCAHO web site at http://www.jointcommission.org/. The JCAHO is an independent, not-for-profit organization that evaluates and accredits more than 15,000 health care organizations and programs in the United States. To receive and maintain JCAHO accreditation, a health care organization must undergo an on-site survey by a JCAHO survey team at least every three years and meet specific standards and performance measurements that affect the safety and quality of patient care.

- **Health Insurance Coverage** - Find out if the physician is covered by your health insurance plan. If you belong to a managed care plan (HMO or PPO), you are usually restricted to using specific physicians who also belong to the Plan. If you decide to use a physician who is "outside the network," you will likely have to pay "out of pocket" for the services provided.

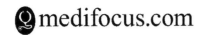

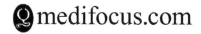medifocus.com

6 - Directory of Organizations

American Association for Pain Management
13947 Mono Way #A; Sonora, CA 95370
209.533.9744   209.533.9750 (fax)
aapm@aapainmanage.org
www.aapainmanage.org

American Chronic Pain Association (ACPA)
POB 850; Rocklin, CA 95677-0850
800.533.3231   916.632.0922; 916.632.3208 (f)
acpa@pacbell.net
www.theacpa.org

American Pain Foundation
201 North Charles Street; Suite 710; Baltimore, MD 21201
888.615.7246   410.783.7292; 410.385.1821 (f)
info@painfoundation.org
www.painfoundation.org

American Pain Society
4700 West Lake Avenue; Glenview, IL 60025
847.375.4715   877.734.8758 (fax)
info@ampainsoc.org
www.ampainsoc.org

American RSDHope
POB 875; Harrison, ME; 04040-0875
207-583-4589
rsdhope@mail.org
www.rsdhope.org

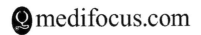
Center for Pain Management; University of Chicago Hospital

5758 S. Maryland Avenue; Chicago, IL 60637
312.842.0200
www.uchospitals.edu/specialties/anesthesia/

International Association for the Study of Pain

111 Queen Anne Avenue Suite 501 Seattle, WA 98109
206.283.0311
iaspdesk@iasp-pain.org
www.iasp-pain.org

International Reflex Sympathetic Dystrophy Foundation

POB 1145; Lakeville, MA 02347
508.946.9888; 508.946.3338 (fax)
www.rsdinfo.com

International Research Foundation for RSD/CRPS

1910 East Busch Blvd. Tampa, FL 33612

813.907-2312
info@rsdfoundation.org
www.rsdfoundation.org

Minnesota RSDS-CRPS Coalition

POB 486; Prior Lake, MN 55372

952.457.7586
rsdsmn@aol.com

National Chronic Pain Outreach Association

POB 274; Millboro, VA 24460
540.862.9437; 540.862.9452 (f)
www.chronicpain.org

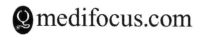

National Foundation for the Treatment of Pain
POB 70045; Houston, TX 77270-0045
713.862.9332; 713.862.9346 (f)
markgordon@paincare.org
www.paincare.org

New York Weill Cornell Medical Center; Pain Medicine Division
1305 York Ave Tenth Floor New York, NY 10021
646.962.7246
www.cornellpainmedicine.org/

PARC (Promoting Awareness of RSD and CRPS in Canada)
POB 21026; St. Catharines, Ontario; L2M 7X2 CANADA
905.934.0261
www.rsdcanada.org

Reflex Sympathetic Dystrophy Syndrome Association
POB 502; Milford, CT 06460
877.662.7737; 203.877.3790
info@rsds.org
www.rsds.org

RSD Alert International
www.rsdalert.co.uk

RSD Fighting Back
Robyn Spicer
jazz@ptdprolog.net
www.rsd-fightingback.org

University of Washington Multidisciplinary Pain Center
1959 NE Pacific; Seattle, WA 98195
206.598.4282
uwmedicine.washington.edu/

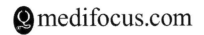

Complementary and Alternative Medicine Resources

American Academy of Medical Acupuncture

170 East Grand Avenue Suite 330 El Segundo, CA 90245 Phone: 310.364.0193
administrato@medicalacupuncture.org
http://www.medicalacupuncture.org

American Association for Acupuncture and Oriental Medicine

1925 West County Road B2
Roseville, MN 55113
Phone: 651.631.0216
http://www.aaaom.edu

American Association of Naturopathic Physicians

4435 Wisconsin Avenue
Suite 403 Washington, DC 20016
Phone (Toll free): 866.538.2267
Phone: 202.237.8150
http://www.naturopathic.org

American Chiropractic Association

1701 Clarendon Blvd.
Arlington, VA 22209
Phone: 703.276.8800 memberinfo@acatoday.org http://www.amerchiro.org

American Holistic Medical Association

23366 Commerce Park Suite 101B Beachwood, OH 44122 Phone: 216.292.6644
info@holisticmedicine.org http://www.holisticmedicine.org

American Massage Therapy Association

500 Davis Street, Suite 900
Evanston, IL 60201-4695
Phone (Toll-Free): 877.905.2700
Phone: 847.864.0123 info@amtamassage.org http://www.amtamassage.org

National Center for Complementary and Alternative Medicine (NCCAM) Clearinghouse

9000 Rockville Pike Bethesda, MD 20892 Phone: 888.644.6226 info@nccam.nih.gov

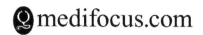

http://nccam.nih.gov

National Center for Homeopathy

801 North Fairfax Street, Suite 306
Alexandria, VA 22314
Phone: 703.548.7790
http://www.homeopathic.org

Office of Dietary Supplements, National Institutes of Health

6100 Executive Boulevard
Room 3B01, MSC 7517
Bethesda, MD 20892-7517
Phone: 301.435.2920 ods@nih.gov http://ods.od.nih.gov

Rosenthal Center for Complementary and Alternative Medicine

Columbia Presbyterian Hospital
630 West 168th Street
Box 75
New York, NY 10032
Phone: 212.342.0101
http://rosenthal.hs.columbia.edu

Made in the USA
Lexington, KY
28 February 2015